EMQs in
CLINICAL
MEDICINE

EMQs in
CLINICAL
MEDICINE

Irfan Syed BSc (Hons), MBBS
PRHO University College Hospital, London &
Royal Sussex County Hospital, Brighton, UK

Editorial Advisors:
Aroon Hingorani MA, FRCP, PhD
BHF Senior Fellow, Reader and Honorary Consultant Physician, BHF
Laboratories, University College London, Centre for Clinical Pharmacology,
Department of Medicine, London, UK

Raymond MacAllister MA, MD, FRCP
Reader in Clinical Pharmacology and Honorary Consultant Physician, BHF
Laboratories, University College London, Centre for Clinical Pharmacology,
Department of Medicine, London, UK

Patrick Vallance BSc (Hons), MD, FRCP, FMedSci
Head, Division of Medicine, Professor of Medicine, University College London,
The Rayne Institute, London, UK

A member of the Hodder Headline Group
LONDON

First published in Great Britain in 2004 by
Arnold, a member of the Hodder Headline Group,
338 Euston Road, London NW1 3BH

http://www.arnoldpublishers.com

Distributed in the United States of America by
Oxford University Press Inc.,
198 Madison Avenue, New York, NY 10016
Oxford is a registered trademark of Oxford University Press

British Library Cataloguing in Publication Data
A catalogue record for this book is available from the British Library

Library of Congress Cataloging-in-Publication Data
A catalog record for this book is available from the Library of Congress

ISBN   0 340 811099

1 2 3 4 5 6 7 8 9 10

Commissioning Editor: Clare Christian & Georgina Bentliff
Project Editor: Heather Smith
Production Controller: Jane Lawrence
Cover Design: Amina Dudhia

Typeset in 9.5/12 Rotis Serif by Charon Tec Pvt. Ltd, Chennai, India.
www.charontec.com
Printed and bound in Malta.

What do you think about this book? Or any other Arnold title?
Please send your comments to **feedback.arnold@hodder.co.uk**

Dedication

To Mum, Dad, Reshma and Zishan

Contents

SECTION 7: METABOLIC AND ENDOCRINE DISTURBANCES   195

SECTION 8: MISCELLANEOUS   213

Preface

Extended matching questions (EMQs) are becoming a more popular means of written assessment in undergraduate and postgraduate medical examinations.

This book provides a set of extended matching questions containing themes that commonly appear in such examinations. Each question section is followed by a concise explanation or additional information about each answer so that you can learn some medicine as well as gaining valuable practice at answering such questions.

Examination technique is an important consideration in answering extended matching questions. The revision boxes aim to train you to pick up on various symptoms/signs/presentations that will, with any luck, improve your chances of choosing the correct answer.

Good luck with your exams!!

Irfan

Acknowledgements

I would like to offer my sincere thanks to Professor Patrick Vallance, Dr Aroon Hingorani and Dr Raymond MacAllister for all their efforts in reviewing and editing the draft of this book. Many thanks are also due to Georgina, Heather, Clare and the staff at Hodder Headline for their efforts in the production of the book.

INTRODUCTION: EMQ REVISION

The most important skill in answering extended matching questions (EMQs) success-fully is picking out important collections of symptoms and/or signs from a question that point to the correct option from the list of options available.

Example

Pulses

A	Mitral stenosis	G	Aortic stenosis
B	Atrial flutter	H	Mitral regurgitation
C	Aortic regurgitation	I	Atrial fibrillation
D	Gaucher's disease	J	Mixed aortic valve disease
E	Acute CO_2 retention	K	Coarctation of aorta
F	Mixed mitral valve disease	L	Cardiac tamponade

For each set of clinical signs, give the most likely cause for the presentation below.

1   Slow rising pulse, narrow pulse pressure, heaving apex beat and fourth heart sound.
G   Angina, shortness of breath, dizziness and syncope on exertion are common presenting symptoms.

Although a slow rising pulse may not be a pathognomonic feature of aortic stenosis it is a highly suggestive feature and the ability to pick out such phrases allows you to answer questions more quickly and with greater success.

The revision boxes are not intended to act as a crash course in the medical specialities described. The aim is to help the reader to identify some typical presenting features, symptoms, signs, investigation results, etc. that crop up in EMQs and are **highly suggestive** of a particular option(s) in the question.

Numbers in squared brackets, e.g. [2], cross-reference parts of the revision box with particular EMQs and explanations from the book.

SECTION 1:
CARDIOVASCULAR
MEDICINE

QUESTIONS

1 Chest pain

A	pulmonary embolus	H	aortic dissection
B	pneumothorax	I	cardiac tamponade
C	lobar pneumonia	J	herpes zoster infection
D	costochondritis	K	tension pneumothorax
E	oesophageal spasm	L	pericarditis
F	atrial fibrillation	M	angina
G	infective endocarditis		

For each clinical presentation below, give the most likely cause for the chest pain. Each option may be used only once.

1   A 63-year-old man with a history of high blood pressure presents in A&E with sudden-onset tearing chest pain radiating to the back

2   A 40-year-old woman develops sudden-onset dyspnoea at rest following hip replacement surgery. On examination she is tachycardic and her electrocardiogram (ECG) shows right axis deviation.

3   A 60-year-old businessman complains of central crushing chest pain radiating to both arms after running to catch a bus. Pain was relieved by rest and his ECG recording 1 h later was unremarkable.

4   A 21-year-old high-jumper presents with acute-onset dyspnoea and right-sided pleuritic chest pain. Examination reveals increased resonance and reduced expansion on the right side.

5   A 23-year-old woman presents with localized left-sided chest pain that is exacerbated by coughing and is particularly painful on light pressure to that area. Pain is relieved by aspirin. The ECG is unremarkable.

Answers: see page 12.

2 Pulses

A	mitral stenosis	G	aortic stenosis
B	atrial flutter	H	mitral regurgitation
C	aortic regurgitation	I	atrial fibrillation
D	Gaucher's disease	J	mixed aortic valve disease
E	acute CO_2 retention	K	coarctation of aorta
F	mixed mitral valve disease	L	cardiac tamponade

For each set of clinical signs, give the most likely cause for the type of pulse felt.

1   Slow rising pulse, narrow pulse pressure, heaving apex beat and fourth heart sound.

2   Collapsing pulse, wide pulse pressure, 'pistol-shot' sound heard over femoral arteries.

3   Radiofemoral delay in a patient with hypertension.

4   Pulsus paradoxus, jugular venous pressure (JVP) rises on inspiration, heart sounds muffled.

5   Bounding pulse in a patient who is short of breath.

Answers: see page 13.

3 Cardiac murmurs

A	mitral stenosis	G	aortic regurgitation
B	atrial flutter	H	tetralogy of Fallot
C	atrial fibrillation	I	atrial septal defect
D	aortic stenosis	J	aortic incompetence
E	friction rub	K	mitral regurgitation
F	tricuspid regurgitation	L	ventricular septal defect

For the following sets of signs, give the most likely cause for the heart murmur. Each option may be used only once.

1 Tapping apex beat, loud S1, mid-diastolic murmur loudest at the apex in expiration lying on the left side.

2 Heaving undisplaced apex beat, absent A2 with ejection systolic murmur radiating to the carotids.

3 Pansystolic murmur heard best at lower left sternal edge during inspiration in a patient with pulsatile hepatomegaly.

4 Displaced, volume-overloaded apex. Soft S1, pansystolic murmur at apex radiating to axilla.

5 Left parasternal heave and harsh pansystolic murmur at lower left sternal edge that is also audible at apex.

Answers: see page 14.

4 Jugular venous pressure

A	tricuspid stenosis	G	complete heart block
B	ventricular fibrillation	H	left heart failure
C	tricuspid regurgitation	I	mitral stenosis
D	constrictive pericarditis	J	aortic stenosis
E	aortic regurgitation	K	superior vena cava obstruction
F	atrial fibrillation	L	normal JVP

For each set of signs give the most likely cause for the particular JVP observed. Each option may be used only once.

1   Elevated JVP with absent pulsation.

2   Giant systolic 'v' waves.

3   Large 'a' waves and slow 'y' descent in JVP. Patient has ascites.

4   Cannon 'a' waves.

5   Raised JVP that rises on inspiration.

Answers: see page 15.

5 ECG abnormalities

A   subendocardial infarction
B   pulmonary embolus
C   right bundle-branch block
D   Mobitz type II second-degree
     heart block
E   hyperkalaemia
F   inferior myocardial infarction
G   anterolateral myocardial
     infarction

H   left bundle-branch block
I   hypokalaemia
J   pericarditis
K   atrial fibrillation
L   mitral regurgitation
M   mitral stenosis

For each clinical scenario/ECG finding give the most likely cause. Each option may be used only once.

1   A 26-year-old woman presents acutely unwell with shortness of breath. Her ECG shows sinus tachycardia, deep S waves in I, inverted T waves in III and Q waves in III.

2   Dominant R in V1, inverted T waves in V1–V3, deep wide S waves in V6.

3   Prolonged P–R interval, depressed ST, flattened T waves, prominent U waves.

4   Sinus rhythm, bifid 'p' waves best seen in II, V3 and V4.

5   A 65-year-old man presents with chest pain radiating to the jaw. The ECG shows ST segment elevation in II, III and aVF, with T-wave inversion in V5 and V6.

Answers: see page 16.

6 ECG abnormalities

A	hyperkalaemia	H	atrial fibrillation
B	mitral regurgitation	I	hypocalcaemia
C	left bundle-branch block	J	atrial flutter
D	normal ECG	K	ventricular tachycardia
E	first-degree heart block	L	right bundle-branch block
F	cardiac tamponade	M	hypokalaemia
G	hypercalcaemia			

For each clinical scenario/ECG finding, give the most likely cause for the clinical findings. Each option may be used only once.

1   ECG of a 55 year old being treated for hypertension shows tall tented T waves.

2   A 34-year-old man presents to A&E after a road traffic accident. The ECG shows pulseless electrical activity.

3   An 85-year-old man with pneumonia complains of palpitations. ECG shows absent P waves.

4   ECG of a 45-year-old man with sarcoidosis shows an 'M' pattern V5 and inverted T waves in I, aVL and V5–V6.

5   ECG of an 8-year-old girl shows normal P waves and QRS complexes but shows T-wave inversion in V1.

Answers: see page 16.

7 Hypertension

A	Cushing's syndrome	G	malignant hypertension
B	systemic sclerosis	H	hyperparathyroidism
C	coarctation of the aorta	I	renal artery stenosis
D	Conn's syndrome	J	portal hypertension
E	pregnancy	K	phaeochromocytoma
F	polycystic kidneys		

For each clinical scenario below, give the most likely cause for the clinical findings. Each option may be used only once.

1   A 30-year-old woman presenting with hypertension is found to have hypokalaemia and a mild metabolic alkalosis.

2   An anxious 26-year-old woman presents with episodes of chest pain and palpitations precipitated by stress and smoking. Her 24-hour urine shows elevated catecholamines.

3   A 45-year-old woman presents with weight gain, muscle weakness and hirsutism. On examination she is hypertensive and has pedal oedema.

4   A 40-year-old man is brought to A&E with severe headache. On examination he has papilloedema and fundal haemorrhages. His BP is 220/145 mmHg.

5   Hypertension in a 75 year old who is a heavy smoker with widespread peripheral vascular disease.

Answers: see page 17.

8 Treatment of heart failure

A nifedipine
B metolazone
C lidnocaine (lignocaine)
D 100 per cent O_2, intravenous diamorphine, intravenous furosemide (frusemide), sublingual glyceryl trinitrate (GTN)
E intravenous isosorbide mononitrate
F digoxin
G 100 per cent O_2, oral diamorphine, oral furosemide (frusemide), intravenous GTN
H intravenous adenosine
I spironolactone
J start cardiopulmonary resuscitation (CPR)
K oral furosemide

For each clinical scenario below, suggest the most appropriate therapy. Each option may be used only once.

1 A 65-year-old man with heart failure requires rate control to treat coexisting atrial fibrillation.

2 A 65-year-old woman being treated with large doses of loop diuretic requires add-on therapy for oedema refractory to treatment.

3 A 69-year-old woman with asthma being treated with a loop diuretic, ACE inhibitor and long-acting nitrate is prescribed a drug to reduce long-term mortality.

4 A 70-year-old woman with a history of chronic heart failure presents with severe pulmonary oedema.

5 Treatment of mild symptoms of shortness of breath and ankle oedema in a 65-year-old man with left ventricular dysfunction caused by ischaemic heart disease. He is already taking an ACE inhibitor.

Answers: see page 18.

9 Treatment of arrhythmias

A	intravenous adenosine	G	low–molecular-weight (LMW) heparin
B	oral warfarin		
C	oral lidocaine (lignocaine)	H	oral amiodarone + warfarin
D	digoxin + warfarin for a month	I	direct current (DC) shock + heparin
E	intravenous magnesium + ventricular pacing		
		J	oral sotalol + warfarin
F	intravenous amiodarone	K	none of the above

For each clinical scenario below, suggest the most appropriate therapy. Each option may be used only once.

1   Treatment of a 65-year-old man with atrial fibrillation (AF) of longer than 48 h before DC cardioversion.

2   Initial therapy in a 60-year-old woman presenting severely compromised with acute persistent AF.

3   A 55-year-old man admitted with an acute myocardial infarction develops a short run of ventricular tachycardia (VT). He requires treatment for prophylaxis against recurrent VT.

4   Drug to aid diagnosis in a 50-year-old man presenting with an unidentifiable, regular, narrow-complex tachycardia.

5   Prophylaxis of ventricular tachycardia in a patient with varying QRS axis and prolonged Q–T interval.

Answers: see page 19.

10 Cardiovascular emergencies

A	oral dobutamine	F	aspirin, heparin
B	DC shock and adrenaline	G	DC shock and atropine
C	100 per cent O$_2$, subcutaneous LMW heparin, intravenous fluids	H	labetalol
		I	emergency renal dialysis
		J	aspirin, GTN
D	nifedipine	K	aspirin, streptokinase
E	atropine		

For each clinical scenario below, suggest the most appropriate therapy. Each option may be used only once.

1   A 57-year-old businessman presents with a 4-h history of crushing chest pain. The ECG changes include ST elevation in II, III and aVF.

2   A 65-year-old man presenting with chest pain becomes unresponsive. His ECG shows ventricular fibrillation.

3   A 40-year-old woman collapses after a flight with breathlessness and right-sided pleuritic chest pain.

4   A 45-year-old man with chronic glomerulonephritis presents with a severe headache. On examination he has papilloedema and bilateral retinal haemorrhages. His BP is 240/132 mmHg.

5   A 55-year-old man requires immediate pharmacological management for severe symptomatic sinus bradycardia.

Answers: see page 21.

ANSWERS

1 Chest pain

Answers: H A M B D

> A 63-year-old man with a history of high blood pressure presents in A&E with sudden-onset tearing chest pain radiating to the back.

H   Pain can also radiate down the arms and into the neck and can be difficult to distinguish from an acute myocardial infarction. Indeed these symptoms are often associated with anterior arch or aortic root dissection. The dissection can interrupt flow to the coronary arteries, resulting in myocardial ischaemia.
The Stanford classification divides dissections into two types: A and B. Type A involves the ascending aorta but type B does not. This system also helps delineate treatment. Usually, type A dissections require surgery, whereas most type B dissections are usually best managed medically by aggressive reduction of blood pressure.

> A 40-year-old woman develops sudden-onset dyspnoea at rest following hip replacement surgery. On examination she is tachycardic and her ECG shows right axis deviation.

A   Patients can also present with signs of hypoxia, pyrexia and later haemoptysis. Look out for risk factors such as recent surgery and immobility in this patient.

> A 60-year-old businessman complains of central crushing chest pain radiating to both arms after running to catch a bus. Pain was relieved by rest and his ECG recording 1 h later was unremarkable.

M   This is a classic description of angina. Pain is usually brought on by exertion but other recognized precipitants include cold weather and emotion.

> A 21-year-old high-jumper presents with acute-onset dyspnoea and right-sided pleuritic chest pain. Examination reveals increased resonance and reduced expansion on the right side.

B   Tall thin young men are especially at risk of having a pneumothorax. The trachea is deviated away from the affected side in a tension pneumothorax. In both simple pneumothorax and tension pneumothorax, expansion is reduced on the affected side. If tension pneumothorax is suspected do not perform a chest radiograph because it may delay emergency treatment. Patients with chronic obstructive pulmonary disease (COPD) are at risk of pneumothorax as a result of bullae rupturing.

A 23-year-old woman presents with localized left-sided chest pain that is exacerbated by coughing and is particularly painful on light pressure to that area. Pain is relieved by aspirin. The ECG is unremarkable.

D   Idiopathic costochondritis is also known as Tietze's syndrome. Localized tenderness to palpation is important for diagnosis. The second rib is frequently affected in this condition.

2 Pulses

Answers: G C K L E

Slow rising pulse, narrow pulse pressure, heaving apex beat and fourth heart sound.

G   Angina, shortness of breath, dizziness and syncope on exertion are common presenting symptoms.

Collapsing pulse, wide pulse pressure, 'pistol-shot' sound heard over femoral arteries.

C   Other signs include Corrigan's sign (carotid pulsation), de Musset's sign (head-nodding) and Quincke's sign (capillary pulsations in nail bed). These are all rare and were described at a time when valve replacement was not available.

Radiofemoral delay in a patient with hypertension.

K   This condition is twice as common in men and involves a narrowing of the aorta. Look out for the association with Turner's syndrome (45XO). A mid to late systolic murmur caused by turbulent flow can sometimes be heard over the upper part of the praecordium. Narrowing of the aorta can result in the formation of a collateral arterial circulation, including the intercostal arteries. These arteries can erode the undersurfaces of ribs, giving rise to notched ribs on chest radiograph.

Pulsus paradoxus, JVP rises on inspiration, heart sounds muffled.

L   The signs of falling blood pressure, rising JVP on inspiration and muffled heart sounds are known as Beck's triad and are an indicator of cardiac tamponade/constrictive pericarditis.

Bounding pulse in a patient who is short of breath.

E   A bounding pulse is a feature of acute rather than chronic CO_2 retention. The mechanism involves reflex vasodilatation to provide adequate tissue perfusion. Hence, a bounding pulse can also be felt in a patient with sepsis (systemic vasodilatation).

3 Cardiac murmurs

Answers: A D F K L

Tapping apex beat, loud S1, mid-diastolic murmur loudest at the apex in expiration lying on the left side.

A   Mitral stenosis is a recognized complication of rheumatic heart disease. Mitral stenosis causing pulmonary hypertension and pulmonary valve regurgitation can result in an early diastolic murmur (Graham–Steell murmur). Mitral stenosis may be associated with symptoms of shortness of breath, chest pain, palpitations and haemoptysis. Atrial fibrillation is also a common finding. Other signs include a malar flush.

Heaving undisplaced apex beat, absent A2 with ejection systolic murmur radiating to the carotids.

D   Aortic stenosis is associated with a narrow pulse pressure and a quiet or absent second heart sound. Symptoms include angina, shortness of breath and syncope. Surgical correction by valve replacement is warranted by the patient's symptoms or the pressure gradient against the valve.

Pansystolic murmur heard best at lower left sternal edge during inspiration in a patient with pulsatile hepatomegaly.

F   Infective endocarditis of the tricuspid valve is a well-recognized cause of tricuspid regurgitation in intravenous drug users. Giant systolic V waves may be seen in the JVP.

Displaced, volume-overloaded apex. Soft S1, pansystolic murmur at apex radiating to axilla.

K   Rheumatic heart disease is still a common cause of mitral regurgitation (MR) in developing countries. Mitral valve prolapse is a more common cause in the USA and western Europe. MR may also develop acutely with myocardial infarction, secondary to papillary muscle rupture, which is often very poorly tolerated. The left ventricle is volume overloaded, increasing left-sided filling pressures and resulting in acute pulmonary oedema and symptoms of dyspnoea.
Rarer causes of MR include the connective tissue diseases, e.g. Marfan's syndrome and Ehlers–Danlos syndrome.

Left parasternal heave and harsh pansystolic murmur at lower left sternal edge that is also audible at apex.

L   Prevalence of ventricular septal defect (VSD) is around 2 in 1000 births. With a small VSD (maladie de Roger) the patient is asymptomatic and treatment is not required (apart from antibiotic prophylaxis against endocarditis for dental work, etc.). Spontaneous closure of the VSD is still possible with larger defects and the complications can be managed medically in the short term, e.g. diuretics to treat heart failure. Indications for surgery include failed medical therapy, growth failure and elevated pulmonary artery pressure.

4 Jugular venous pressure

Answers: K C A G D

Elevated JVP with absent pulsation.

K Bronchial carcinoma is a well-recognized cause of this medical emergency. Symptoms include early morning headache (feeling of fullness in the head) and signs include facial congestion and oedema involving the upper limb.
Either radiotherapy or chemotherapy may be useful depending on the sensitivity of the tumour type.

Giant systolic 'v' waves.

C Tricuspid regurgitation is associated with giant systolic V waves. The V wave represents regurgitant blood ejected from the right ventricle at systole.

Large 'a' waves and slow 'y' descent in JVP. Patient has ascites.

A Rheumatic fever is the most common cause of tricuspid stenosis. There is usually involvement of other valves, e.g. coexisting mitral stenosis. The prominent symptom is fatigue. The presence of shortness of breath suggests concomitant mitral valve disease.
Surgical intervention by tricuspid valve replacement is usually carried out only when there are other defective valves also being operated on.

Cannon 'a' waves.

G Cannon waves occur when there is atrioventricular (AV) dissociation. The classic example is complete heart block but it may also be seen in ventricular tachycardia, and in patients with a single chamber pacemaker and continuing atrial contractions. This is rare nowadays because such patients are invariably given dual-chamber pacemakers. The cannon wave is generated by the atrium contracting in the presence of a closed tricuspid valve resulting from simultaneous ventricular systole.

Raised JVP that rises on inspiration.

D Kussmaul's sign refers to the paradoxical rising of the JVP with inspiration. This sign can also be observed in cardiac tamponade. Usually the JVP falls as a result of the rise in intrathoracic pressure during inspiration.

5 ECG abnormalities

Answers: B C I M F

A 26-year-old woman presents acutely unwell with shortness of breath. Her ECG shows sinus tachycardia, deep S waves in I, inverted T waves in III and Q waves in III.

B This is the S I, Q III, T III pattern frequently quoted in books but it is actually rare in practice. Right axis deviation may be present but the ECG is often normal in small/medium pulmonary emboli.

Dominant R in V1, inverted T waves in V1–V3, deep wide S waves in V6.

C The 'MARROW' pattern, e.g. 'RSR' pattern in V1 (M) with deep wide S wave in V6 (W). Causes include atrial septal defect (ASD) and pulmonary embolus.

Prolonged P–R interval, depressed ST, flattened T waves, prominent U waves.

I Look out for loop/thiazide diuretics as a cause of hypokalaemia.

Sinus rhythm, bifid 'p' waves best seen in II, V3 and V4.

M Known as P mitrale, this bifid P wave suggests left atrial hypertrophy. A peaked P wave is called P pulmonale and suggests right atrial hypertrophy.

A 65-year-old man presents with chest pain radiating to the jaw. The ECG shows ST segment elevation in II, III and aVF, with T-wave inversion in V5 and V6.

F Anterolateral MI would involve leads related to that portion of the heart, e.g. V4–V6, I, aVL.

6 ECG abnormalities

Answers: A F H C D

ECG of a 55 year old being treated for hypertension shows tall tented T waves.

A Look out for potassium-sparing diuretics and angiotensin-converting enzyme (ACE) inhibitors as a cause. Other causes include renal failure and metabolic acidosis.

A 34-year-old man presents to A&E after a road traffic accident. The ECG shows pulseless electrical activity.

F Pulseless electrical activity (PEA) is a clinical condition characterized by loss of a palpable pulse in the presence of recordable cardiac electrical activity. PEA is also referred to as electromechanical dissociation (EMD). Given the history of trauma in this question, cardiac tamponade is the most likely cause.

Management of PEA should follow current advanced life support guidelines while possible reversible causes are sought.

An 85-year-old man with pneumonia complains of palpitations. ECG shows absent P waves.

H   Absent P waves is the classic ECG finding of atrial fibrillation. This condition is associated with a significantly increased risk of an embolic event, e.g. stroke. Remember that hyperthyroidism is a cause of atrial fibrillation and thyroid function tests are indicated on first presentation. Uncontrolled atrial fibrillation is associated with an irregularly irregular pulse. An echocardiogram is useful to detect any existing structural abnormalities such as left atrial enlargement caused by mitral valve disease.

ECG of a 45-year-old man with sarcoidosis shows an 'M' pattern V5 and inverted T waves in I, aVL and V5–V6.

C   Left bundle-branch block (LBBB) is associated with the 'WILLIAM' pattern, e.g. 'M' pattern in V5. In LBBB, there is conduction of impulse from the right ventricle to the interventricular septum, and then to the anterior and posterior portions of the left ventricle before it finally reaches the left lateral free wall. Delayed left ventricular depolarization is responsible for the ECG findings in LBBB.

ECG of an 8-year-old girl shows normal P waves and QRS complexes but shows T-wave inversion in V1.

D   T inversion is a normal finding in leads V1–V3 in children.

7 Hypertension

Answers: D K A G I

A 30-year-old woman presenting with hypertension is found to have hypokalaemia and a mild metabolic alkalosis.

D   The combination of hypertension, hypokalaemia and metabolic alkalosis is suggestive of primary hyperaldosteronism. This is usually caused by Conn's syndrome (unilateral adrenocortical adenoma) or bilateral adrenal hyperplasia. This is a rare cause of secondary hypertension but is more common in young people with hypertension.

An anxious 26-year-old woman presents with episodes of chest pain and palpitations precipitated by stress and smoking. Her 24-hour urine shows elevated catecholamines.

K   Phaeochromocytoma is a catecholamine-secreting tumour and is very rare. Symptoms, including palpitations, tachycardia, anxiety and blanching, are non-specific and may be misdiagnosed. A patient may present as a medical emergency with a hypertensive crisis. The ECG usually reveals left ventricular hypertrophy.
      Rarely, phaeochromocytoma can be inherited in an autosomal dominant fashion as multiple endocrine neoplasia (MEN) type IIa (includes medullary thyroid carcinoma, parathyroid hyperplasia).

A 45-year-old woman presents with weight gain, muscle weakness and hirsutism. On examination she is hypertensive and has pedal oedema.

A   These are symptoms of chronic glucocorticoid excess. Other symptoms include menstrual irregularities and mood disturbance. Causes of Cushing's syndrome include administration of exogenous steroids, ACTH-secreting pituitary tumours and adrenal adenomas (see Question 78, p. 203).

A 40-year-old man is brought to A&E with severe headache. On examination he has papilloedema and fundal haemorrhages. His BP is 220/145 mmHg.

G   Malignant hypertension is severe hypertension associated with acute end-organ failure, e.g. encephalopathy, renal failure. By definition there must be grade III–IV hypertensive changes.
      Treatment involves careful reduction in blood pressure over several days, usually with oral therapy. Care should be taken to avoid precipitous reduction in blood pressure because this may lead to watershed infarction.

Hypertension in a 75 year old who is a heavy smoker with widespread peripheral vascular disease.

I   Renal disease is the most common cause of secondary hypertension. Intrinsic renal disease, e.g. glomerulonephritis, makes up most of these cases. Renal artery stenosis is responsible for around 25 per cent of all cases of renal hypertension Treatment is directed at reducing blood pressure and preserving renal function. Revascularization may be performed but there is no consensus as to which patients may benefit from this therapy compared with from medical treatment.

8 Treatment of heart failure

Answers: F B I D K

A 65-year-old man with heart failure requires rate control to treat coexisting atrial fibrillation.

F   Digoxin has a narrow therapeutic window and toxicity with normal doses can be precipitated by hypokalaemia, hypomagnesaemia, renal impairment and hypercalcaemia. Signs of digoxin toxicity include confusion, nausea, arrhythmias and visual disturbance.

A 65-year-old woman being treated with large doses of loop diuretic requires add-on therapy for oedema refractory to treatment.

B   Thiazides may be added to loop diuretics in resistant oedema because they have a synergistic mechanism of action. Metolazone is often the drug of choice because it remains effective even in the presence of significant renal impairment.

A 69-year-old woman with asthma being treated with a loop diuretic, ACE inhibitor and long-acting nitrate is prescribed a drug to reduce long-term mortality.

I   Spironolactone was shown to decrease long-term mortality when added to conventional therapy in the RALES (Randomised Aldactone Evaluation Study) trial. This double-masked study* enrolled patients with severe heart failure (no more than 35 per cent ejection fraction), randomizing them to daily spironolactone/placebo. The trial was discontinued early as a result of the finding of a 30 per cent reduction in the risk of death in the spironolactone group.

A 70-year-old woman with a history of chronic heart failure presents with severe pulmonary oedema.

D   Acute pulmonary oedema is a life-threatening medical emergency and the diuretic should be given parenterally. Elderly patients may suffer from COPD/asthma or have a coexisting chest infection and should therefore be given antibiotics and nebulized bronchodilators as required.

Treatment of mild symptoms of shortness of breath and ankle oedema in a 65-year-old man with left ventricular dysfunction caused by ischaemic heart disease. He is already taking an ACE inhibitor.

K   Patients with mild left ventricular dysfunction may be satisfactorily controlled on an ACE inhibitor. If, however, shortness of breath and ankle oedema are not sufficiently controlled, oral diuretics are added. The drug of choice is a loop diuretic.

9 Treatment of arrhythmias

Answers: D I F A E

Treatment of a 65-year-old man with AF of longer than 48 h before DC cardioversion.

* Pitt *et al. New England Journal of Medicine* 1999; **341** 709–17

D   A patient with AF of longer than 48 h duration is at risk of thromboembolism after cardioversion. Unless the patient is severely compromised, it is standard practice to anticoagulate the patient with warfarin for a month before attempting elective cardioversion. During that time the ventricular rate is controlled by prescribing digoxin.

Initial therapy in a 60-year-old woman presenting severely compromised with acute persistent AF.

I   In this case immediate DC shock is indicated because the patient is severely compromised. The administration of heparin decreases but does not abolish the risk of thromboembolism after cardioversion.

A 55-year-old man admitted with an acute myocardial infarction develops a short run of VT. He requires treatment for prophylaxis against recurrent VT.

F   Amiodarone has class I, II, III and IV actions but is used clinically for its class III actions. Class III drugs prolong the plateau phase of the cardiac action potential and increase the absolute refractory period. As a consequence they also prolong the Q–T interval.
Amiodarone is the drug of choice to treat VT. When it is used chronically it has a number of adverse effects but these are not an issue in the acute scenario. These adverse effects include bradycardia, pulmonary fibrosis, hepatic fibrosis, corneal microdeposits (regress if drug is stopped), photosensitive rash and thyroid dysfunction.

Drug to aid diagnosis in a 50-year-old man presenting with an unidentifiable, regular, narrow-complex tachycardia.

A   Adenosine causes profound short-term AV block. In this way it can be used to terminate tachycardias involving an AV re-entry circuit. It may also be used in the diagnosis of an unidentified arrhythmia. Adenosine can cause bronchoconstriction and stimulates nociceptive afferent neurons in the heart. The patient should be warned in advance that he may experience symptoms of chest pain after the drug is administered.

Prophylaxis of ventricular tachycardia in a patient with varying QRS axis and prolonged Q–T interval.

E   This is torsades de points, which will often degenerate to ventricular fibrillation leading to cardiac arrest. Causes include drugs, electrolyte disturbance and congenital long Q–T syndrome. Conventional anti-arrhythmics will make this condition worse.
The treatment of choice is intravenous magnesium sulphate and ventricular pacing at a high rate.

10 Cardiovascular emergencies

Answers: K B C H E

> A 57-year-old businessman presents with a 4-h history of crushing chest pain. The ECG changes include ST elevation in II, III and aVF.

K   This is the presentation of an inferior myocardial infarction and thrombolysis is indicated. Streptokinase is effective in reducing mortality when it is given early, ideally within a few hours of the onset of the chest pain. Contraindications for thrombolysis include any form of internal bleeding, pregnancy, recent head trauma, cerebral malignancy, acute pancreatitis, recent haemorrhagic stroke and oesophageal varices. In these cases urgent primary angioplasty may be deemed a viable alternative.

> A 65-year-old man presenting with chest pain becomes unresponsive. His ECG shows ventricular fibrillation.

B   DC shock is indicated according to current ACLS (Advanced Cardiac Life Support) guidelines, which emphasize the importance of early defibrillation. Defibrillation should not be delayed to give adrenaline, which should be administered if three shocks (200 J, 200 J, 360 J) have been unsuccessful/contraindicated.

> A 40-year-old woman collapses after a flight with breathlessness and right-sided pleuritic chest pain.

C   This is a presentation of pulmonary embolus (PE). Streptokinase has also been used successfully following a major embolism. Open embolectomy is indicated following a massive PE if thrombolysis is unsuccessful/contraindicated.

> A 45-year-old man with chronic glomerulonephritis presents with a severe headache. On examination he has papilloedema and bilateral retinal haemorrhages. His BP is 240/132 mmHg.

H   This is the presentation of malignant hypertension. The therapeutic aim should be rapid, but gradual and controllable reduction in blood pressure is the ideal. Both oral and parenteral therapy may be used depending on the clinician's preference. Sublingual nifedipine is contraindicated because it may produce a profound uncontrollable reduction in the patient which may compromise cerebral perfusion.

> A 55-year-old man requires immediate pharmacological management for severe symptomatic sinus bradycardia.

E   Atropine is the drug of choice. It is a muscarinic acetylcholine receptor antagonist and thus increases the heart rate by inhibiting vagal tone of the heart. If the patient does not respond to atropinization, cardiac pacing should be instituted.

REVISION BOXES

Cardiovascular medicine

These descriptions of pulses in an extended matching question (EMQ) are highly suggestive of the conditions described (Box 1).

Box 1   Conditions indicated by pulses [2]

Pulse	Condition
Irregularly irregular	Atrial fibrillation
Slow-rising pulse	Aortic stenosis
Collapsing pulse	Aortic regurgitation
Bounding pulse	Acute CO_2 retention, hepatic failure, sepsis
Radiofemoral delay	Coarctation of aorta
Jerky pulse	Hypertrophic obstructive cardiomyopathy
	Mitral regurgitation
Pulsus bisferiens	Mixed aortic valve disease
	Hypertrophic obstructive cardiomyopathy
Pulsus paradoxus	Constrictive pericarditis
	Cardiac tamponade

The descriptions of the jugular venous pressure (JVP) in Box 2, often given in an EMQ, are highly suggestive of the conditions described.

Box 2   Conditions indicated by jugular venous pressure [4]

JVP	Condition
Raised, fixed JVP	Superior vena cava obstruction
JVP rising on inspiration	Cardiac tamponade
	Constrictive pericarditis
Large 'v' waves	Tricuspid regurgitation
Absent 'a' waves	Atrial fibrillation
Cannon 'a' waves	Complete heart block
	Atrioventricular (AV) dissociation
	Ventricular arrhythmias

Descriptions of a murmur that require you to detect a valvular defect or other cardiac anomaly are common in EMQs (Box 3).

Box 3 Murmurs and heart sounds [3]

Mitral stenosis	Aortic regurgitation
• Tapping apex beat • Loud first heart sound • Rumbling mid-diastolic murmur at apex (louder in left lateral position on expiration)	• Wide pulse pressure • Displaced, volume-overloaded apex beat • Early diastolic murmur at lower sternal edge (best heard in expiration leaning forward)
Mitral regurgitation	**Tricuspid regurgitation**
• Displaced, volume overloaded apex beat • Soft first heart sound • Pansystolic murmur at apex radiating to axilla (louder in expiration)	• Large systolic 'v' waves • Pansystolic murmur lower left sternal edge (best heard in inspiration)
Aortic stenosis	**Ventricular septal defect**
• Narrow pulse pressure • Heaving undisplaced apex beat • Soft second heart sound • Ejection systolic murmur heard in aortic area radiating to carotids and apex	• Harsh pansystolic murmur lower left sternal edge • Left parasternal heave

If you find any of the physical signs in Box 4 in a cardiology EMQ, look out for the corresponding condition stated in the options. It is likely to be the correct answer!!

Box 4 Physical signs associated with cardiac conditions

Physical sign	Condition
Malar (cheek) flush	Mitral stenosis
Pulsatile hepatomegaly	Tricuspid regurgitation
Carotid pulsation (Corrigan's sign)	Aortic regurgitation
Head nodding (De Musset's sign)	Aortic regurgitation
Capillary pulsations in nail-bed (Quincke's sign)	Aortic regurgitation
Pistol-shot heard over femorals (Traube's sign)	Aortic regurgitation
Roth's spots (boat-shaped retinal haemorrhages)	Infective endocarditis
Osler's nodes (painful hard swellings on fingers/toes)	Infective endocarditis
Janeway's lesions (painless erythematous blanching macules seen on palmar surface)	Infective endocarditis

You should particularly look out for congenital heart defects if the scenario concerns a child.

Box 5 highlights some features of congenital heart defects that may appear in EMQs.

Box 5 Congenital heart defects

Symptoms/signs	Congenital heart defects
• Wide, fixed split second heart sound Ejection systolic murmur second, third intercostal space	Atrial septal defect
• Harsh pansystolic murmur left sternal edge	Ventricular septal defect
• Radiofemoral delay, hypertension	Coarctation of aorta
• Continuous 'machinery' murmur below left clavicle	Persistent ductus arteriosus
• Cyanosis first day of life Chest radiograph: egg-shaped ventricles	Transposition great vessels
• Cyanosis first month of life Chest radiograph: boot-shaped heart	Tetralogy of Fallot

Box 6 summarizes some examples of causes of various ECG findings that may crop up in EMQs. An EMQ may require you to localize an infarct. Box 7 may help you to do this.

Box 6 ECG findings [5, 6]

ECG findings	Condition
• 'Saw-tooth' pattern with normal complexes	Atrial flutter
• Absent 'p' wave	Atrial fibrillation Sinoatrial block
• Bifid 'p' wave	Left atrial hypertrophy, e.g. mitral stenosis
• Peaked 'p' wave	Right atrial hypertrophy, e.g. pulmonary hypertension, tricuspid stenosis
• ST depression	Myocardial ischaemia
• ST elevation	Acute myocardial infarction (MI) Left ventricular aneurysm
• 'Saddle'-shaped ST elevation	Acute constrictive pericarditis
• S I, Q III, T III pattern (deep S waves in I, Q waves in III, inverted T waves in III)	Pulmonary embolus
• Tall tented 't' waves, wide QRS complex (sine wave)	Hyperkalaemia
• Flattened 't' waves, prominent 'U' waves (muscle weakness, cramps, tetany)	Hypokalaemia
• Long 'Q–T' interval, tetany, perioral paraesthesia, carpopedal spasm	Hypocalcaemia

Box 7 Myocardial infarction: ECG changes [5, 6]

ECG changes	Type of MI
Hyperacute T waves (inverts later), ST elevation and then Q wave formation; Localizing infarct (leads with above ECG changes):	
II, III, aVF	Inferior infarct
I, aVL, V2–V6	Anterolateral infarct
V2-V5	Anterior infarct
ST and T wave changes but no Q waves	Subendocardial infarct
Reciprocal changes V1, V2 (tall R waves, ST depression, tall upright T waves)	Posterior infarct

In exam EMQs certain cardiovascular drugs tend to be associated with particular side effects (Box 8).

Box 8 Side effects associated with cardiovascular drugs

Side effect	Drug

• Impotence
  Shortness of breath
  Cold peripheries
	β blockers, e.g. propranolol

• Persistent dry cough	ACE (angiotensin-converting enzyme) inhibitor, e.g. captopril
• Gynaecomastia	Digoxin, spironolactone

• Hyper-/hypothyroidism
  Corneal microdeposits
  Lung/liver fibrosis
	Amiodarone

• Constipation	Verapamil
• Flushing, headache, ankle oedema	Nifedipine
• Gout (hyperuricaemia)	Thiazide diuretic, e.g. bendrofluazide
• Increased hair growth	Minoxidil
• Drug-induced systemic lupus erythematosus (SLE)	Hydralazine

SECTION 2: RESPIRATORY MEDICINE

QUESTIONS

11 Shortness of breath

A   pleural effusion
B   pulmonary oedema
C   right–sided rib fracture
D   pneumothorax
E   bronchogenic carcinoma
F   pneumonia
G   fibrosing alveolitis

H   extrinsic allergic alveolitis
I   anaemia
J   pulmonary embolus
K   acute respiratory distress
    syndrome
L   cystic fibrosis

For each clinical scenario below, give the most likely cause for the clinical findings. Each option may be used only once.

1   A 21-year-old man has a productive cough, wheeze and steatorrhoea. On examination he is clubbed and cyanosed, and has bilateral coarse crackles.

2   A 63-year-old man presents to A&E with weight loss, cough, haemoptysis and shortness of breath. On examination he is anaemic, clubbed and apyrexial.

3   A 65-year-old man presents with shortness of breath and cough productive of pink frothy sputum. On examination he is cyanosed and tachycardic, and has bibasal end-inspiratory crackles. His jugular venous pressure (JVP) is elevated.

4   A 70-year-old woman presents with fever, rigors, shortness of breath and right-sided pleuritic chest pain. On examination the right side of the chest shows reduced expansion, dull percussion and increased tactile vocal fremitus.

5   A 30-year-old farmer presents with repeated episodes of fever, rigors, dry cough and shortness of breath with onset several hours after starting work. On examination he is pyrexial with coarse end-expiratory crackles. His chest radiograph shows mid-zone mottling.

Answers: see page 37.

12 Causes of pneumonia

A	*Legionella pneumophila*	H	*Mycoplasma pneumoniae*
B	*Aspergillus fumigatus*	I	*Escherichia coli*
C	*Pneumocystis carinii*	J	*Chlamydia pneumoniae*
D	*Streptococcus pneumoniae*	K	*Moraxella catarrhalis*
E	cytomegalovirus (CMV) infection	L	varicella zoster
F	*Chlamydia psittaci*	M	*Staphylococcus aureus*
G	*Coxiella burnettii*	N	*Pseudomonas* sp.

For each presentation of pneumonia, choose the most likely infective cause. Each option may be used only once.

1   An 80-year-old man presents with bilateral cavitating bronchopneumonia after an influenza infection.

2   A 24-year-old student presents with severe headache, fever, dry cough and arthralgia. He has recently bought several parrots and was previously fit and well.

3   A 40-year-old man with HIV presents with fever, dry cough, weight loss and exertional dyspnoea.

4   A 75-year-old man presents with headache, dry cough, anaemia and a skin rash. Blood tests detect cold agglutinins.

5   A 25-year-old air-conditioning technician, who suffered from flu-like symptoms a week ago, has developed a dry cough. His chest radiograph shows multilobar shadowing. Blood tests show hyponatraemia and lymphopenia. Urinalysis reveals haematuria.

Answers: see page 38.

13 Haemoptysis

A	tuberculosis (TB)	G	Goodpasture's syndrome
B	haemothorax	H	haemophilia
C	bronchogenic carcinoma	I	pulmonary oedema
D	polyarteritis nodosa	J	pneumonia
E	Wegener's granulomatosis	K	pulmonary embolus
F	bronchiectasis	L	Churg–Strauss syndrome

For each clinical scenario below, give the most likely cause for the clinical findings. Each option may be used only once.

1   A 65-year-old smoker presents with shortness of breath, gallop rhythm and production of pink frothy sputum.

2   A 24-year-old man initially complaining of cough and intermittent haemoptysis presents a few weeks later with haematuria. Biopsy confirms a crescentic glomerulonephritis. Renal biopsy shows linear pattern deposition on immunofluorescence.

3   A 34-year-old woman originally complaining of nasal obstruction develops cough, haemoptysis and pleuritic chest pain. Her chest radiograph shows multiple nodular masses.

4   A 22-year-old man presents with fever, nightsweats, weight loss and cough productive of cupfuls of blood. Ziehl–Neelsen stain is positive for acid-fast bacilli.

5   A 35-year-old businessman returns from a trip abroad and collapses at the airport with haemoptysis and pleuritic chest pain. He has a sinus tachycardia and his ECG shows right axis deviation.

Answers: see page 39.

14 Chest radiograph pathology

A	mitral stenosis	H	right lower lobe collapse
B	bronchiectasis	I	Wegener's granulomatosis
C	right upper lobe collapse	J	Caplan's syndrome
D	Kartagener's syndrome	K	post-fracture fat embolus
E	aortic stenosis	L	right ventricular failure
F	previous varicella pneumonitis	M	left ventricular failure
G	asbestosis			

For each description of a chest radiograph below, give the most likely cause for observed markings. Each option may be used only once.

1 Multiple bilateral nodules between 0.5 and 5 cm in a former miner with rheumatoid arthritis.

2 Kerley B lines, bat-wing shadowing, prominent upper lobe vessels, cardiomegaly.

3 Trachea deviated to right, horizontal fissure and right hilum displaced upwards.

4 Numerous calcified nodules sized less than 5 mm located predominantly in the lower zones of the lungs.

5 Double shadow right heart border, prominent left atrial appendage, left main bronchus elevation.

Answers: see page 41.

15 Chest radiograph pathology

A pneumonia
B silicosis
C bronchiectasis
D aspergillosis
E mesothelioma
F cryptogenic fibrosing
   alveolitis

G chronic obstructive pulmonary
   disease (COPD)
H carcinoma of bronchus
I tuberculosis
J berylliosis
K sarcoidosis
M extrinsic allergic alveolitis

For each scenario below, give the most likely cause for the clinical findings. Each option may be used only once.

1   A 28-year-old African–Caribbean man presents with dry cough and progressive shortness of breath. His chest radiograph shows bilateral hilar lymphadenopathy.

2   The chest radiograph of a 13-year-old boy with cystic fibrosis has tramline and ring shadows.

3   A 65-year-old dockyard worker presents with weight loss and shortness of breath. He is clubbed and cachectic. His chest radiograph shows pleural calcification and a lobulated pleural mass.

4   A 40-year-old woman presents with gross clubbing and progressive shortness of breath. Examination reveals fine end-inspiratory crackles. Her chest radiograph shows a ground-glass appearance of the lung.

5   A 65-year-old smoker presents with shortness of breath. On the chest radiograph, eight ribs can be seen anteriorly above the diaphragm on each side of the chest in the mid-clavicular line.

Answers: see page 42.

16 Treatment of asthma and COPD

A	low–dose oral aminophylline	H	inhaled salmeterol
B	oral prednisolone	I	home 100 per cent oxygen
C	inhaled beclomethasone	J	inhaled aminophylline
D	inhaled ipratropium bromide	K	inhaled salbutamol
E	nebulized ipratropium bromide	M	oral sodium cromoglycate
F	inhaled sodium cromoglycate	N	inhaled salbutamol with spacer
G	nebulized salbutamol		

For each clinical scenario below, suggest the most appropriate therapy. Each option may be used only once.

1   A 7-year-old girl with slight wheeze and shortness of breath despite inhaled salbutamol.

2   A 22-year-old student with mild asthma that needs treatment for occasional early morning wheeze.

3   A 17-year-old student complains that he has to use his salbutamol inhaler regularly to control wheezing.

4   A 32-year-old patient taking maximum dose-inhaled therapy and slow-release theophylline shows persistently inadequate control of symptoms.

5   A 25-year-old woman requires add-on therapy because inhaled beclomethasone and salbutamol do not adequately combat her symptoms.

Answers: see page 43.

17 Emergency management: respiratory distress

A   intubation
B   left-sided decompression
C   chest radiograph
D   nasal intermittent positive
    pressure ventilation
E   28 per cent O_2, nebulized salbu-
    tamol, oral prednisolone
F   emergency tracheostomy
G   28 per cent O_2, nebulized salbu-
    tamol, intramuscular adrenaline
H   right-sided decompression
I   28 per cent O_2, nebulized
    salbutamol, intravenous
    hydrocortisone
J   chest drain
K   100 per cent O_2, intramuscular
    adrenaline, nebulized salbutamol
L   intravenous hydrocortisone
M   100 per cent O_2, nebulized
    salbutamol, intravenous
    hydrocortisone

For each clinical scenario below, suggest the most appropriate intervention. Each option may be used only once.

1   A 65-year-old man with long-standing COPD presents with severe shortness of breath. He has been treated with oxygen and nebulized bronchodilators. An hour later: PaO_2 6.0 kPa (on max. O_2), $PaCO_2$ 16.0 kPa, pH 7.2.

2   A 17-year-old woman presents with wheeze and marked perioral swelling: PaO_2 7.0 kPa (on 28 per cent O_2), $PaCO_2$ 4.1 kPa.

3   A 14 year old with asthma presents with an acute severe asthma attack. PaO_2 10.0 kPa (on 28 per cent O_2), $PaCO_2$ 8.0 kPa.

4   A 28-year-old man involved in a road traffic accident presents with severe respiratory distress. Examination reveals decreased expansion on the right side of the chest with mediastinal shift to the left.

5   A young man presents with an acute onset shortness of breath. Examination reveals decreased expansion on the right: SaO_2 95 per cent.

Answers: see page 44.

18 Management of COPD

A   inhaled salbutamol
B   60 per cent O_2 nebulized salbu-
    tamol, oral prednisolone, oral
    amoxicillin
C   intravenous salbutamol
D   long-term O_2 therapy
E   lung transplantation
F   28 per cent O_2, nebulized salbu-
    tamol + ipratropium, oral
    prednisolone, oral amoxicillin

G   28 per cent O_2, inhaled
    bronchodilators, intravenous
    amoxicillin
H   oral aminophylline
I   ICU admission and intubation
J   100 per cent O_2, amoxicillin
K   intravenous salmeterol
L   NIPPV

For each clinical scenario below, suggest the most appropriate therapy. Each
option may be used only once.

1   A previously healthy 65-year-old smoker with early COPD complains of
    shortness of breath on exertion.

2   A 65-year-old woman with longstanding COPD presents with shortness of
    breath and cough productive of coloured sputum.

3   A 70-year-old man admitted with acute severe exacerbation of COPD does not
    respond to oxygen and nebulized bronchodilators.

4   A 65-year-old patient with advanced COPD treated with bronchodilators and
    steroids still feels breathless. His baseline PaO_2 is around 6.5 kPa.

5   A 55-year-old patient with COPD requires regular add-on therapy after
    bronchodilators do not control symptoms.

Answers: see page 46.

19 Treatment of respiratory infections

A   intravenous benzylpenicillin
B   oral flucloxacillin
C   oral tetracycline
D   oral ciprofloxacin
E   intravenous ceftazidime
F   oral isoniazid + rifampicin
G   intravenous flucloxacillin
H   oral amoxicillin

I   high–dose AZT
     (zidovudine) + pyrazinamide
J   intravenous amoxicillin
K   intravenous co-trimoxazole
L   intravenous teicoplanin
M   intravenous
     cefuroxime + erythromycin

For each clinical scenario below, suggest the most appropriate management. Each option may be used only once.

1   Standard therapy for community-acquired pneumococcal pneumonia not requiring hospital admission.

2   A 35-year-old patient on the ward admitted to hospital 10 days ago presents with severe pneumonia.

3   A 40-year-old builder presents with a severe community-acquired pneumonia. Atypical pathogens are suspected.

4   A 22-year-old HIV-positive individual on anti-retroviral therapy presents with *Pneumocystis carinii* pneumonia.

5   A 19-year-old man contracts pneumonia with symptoms of headache, fever and dry cough. Serology shows evidence of chlamydia infection.

Answers: see page 47.

ANSWERS

11 Shortness of breath

Answers: L E B F H

> A 21-year-old man has a productive cough, wheeze and steatorrhoea. On examination he is clubbed and cyanosed, and has bilateral coarse crackles.

L   Cystic fibrosis is an autosomal recessive condition associated with a mutation in the *CFTR* (cystic fibrosis transmembrane conductance regulator) gene on chromosome 7.
     Patients are susceptible to recurrent respiratory infection and the development of bronchiectasis. Acute exacerbations are often caused by *Pseudomonas* spp. which may be highly resistant to antibiotics. Haemoptysis is common and may indicate the presence of aspergilloma. Pancreatic insufficiency usually develops resulting in malabsorption and steatorrhoea. Growth and puberty are delayed in most patients. Males are usually infertile as a result of the failure of the vas deferens and epididymis to develop. High sweat sodium and chloride concentrations (>60 mmol/l) are highly suggestive of the disease.

> A 63-year-old man presents to A&E with weight loss, cough, haemoptysis and shortness of breath. On examination he is anaemic, clubbed and apyrexial.

E   Remember respiratory causes of clubbing: carcinoma of the bronchus, mesothelioma, bronchiectasis, abscess, empyema, cryptogenic fibrosing alveolitis and cystic fibrosis. COPD and asthma are not causes of clubbing.

> A 65-year-old man presents with shortness of breath and cough productive of pink frothy sputum. On examination he is cyanosed and tachycardic, and has bibasal end-inspiratory crackles. His JVP is elevated.

B   This is the presentation of acute pulmonary oedema secondary to left ventricular failure. Pulmonary oedema occurs because left-sided filling pressures are elevated, causing high pulmonary capillary pressures. This results in transudation of fluid from the plasma into the alveoli, impairing gas exchange and reducing pulmonary compliance. Sputum is often pink as a result of leakage of red blood cells into the alveoli which is a consequence of ruptured pulmonary capillaries.

> A 70-year-old woman presents with fever, rigors, shortness of breath and right-sided pleuritic chest pain. On examination the right side of the chest shows reduced expansion, dull percussion and increased tactile vocal fremitus

F   Reduced expansion, dullness to percussion and increased tactile vocal fremitus, in combination, suggest consolidation. Bronchial breathing is also a feature of consolidation and results from transmission of airway sounds through the consolidated lung to the periphery.
Strictly speaking, consolidation refers to the replacement of alveolar air by fluid, cells, tissue or other material. The most common cause is pneumonia.

A 30-year-old farmer presents with repeated episodes of fever, rigors, dry cough and shortness of breath with onset several hours after starting work. On examination he is pyrexial with coarse end-expiratory crackles. His chest radiograph shows mid-zone mottling.

H   This is a classic presentation of extrinsic allergic alveolitis (EAA), which is a hypersensitivity reaction to inhaled antigens. In farmers, the antigen often responsible is thermophilic actinomycetes in mouldy hay or *Aspergillus clavatus* on germinating barley.
Lung function tests reveal a reversible restrictive defect. The cause of the reaction may be determined by finding serum-precipitating antibodies. In chronic EAA a honeycomb lung can sometimes be seen on the chest radiograph. Acute cases may be treated with corticosteroids but allergen avoidance is the key preventive measure.

12 Causes of pneumonia

Answers: M F C H A

An 80-year-old man presents with bilateral cavitating bronchopneu-monia after an influenza infection.

M   Although not a common pathogen in community-acquired pneumonia, *Staphylococcus aureus* may cause pneumonia in debilitated patients, including elderly people and those recovering from influenza. It is also seen in intravenous drug users (IVDUs) as a consequence of haematological seeding from infected needles, often in association with staphylococcal endocarditis of the tricuspid valve. Flucloxacillin is the treatment of choice for staphylococcal infection.

A 24-year-old student presents with severe headache, fever, dry cough and arthralgia. He has recently bought several parrots and was previously fit and well.

F   Psittacosis is a rare cause of community-acquired pneumonia. It should be suspected in any patient presenting with lower respiratory tract symp-toms and signs who has a history of exposure to birds. No acute diag-nostic tests are available and diagnosis is made in retrospect by demonstrating a rising titre of complement-fixing antibody. As with other atypical cases of pneumonia such as *Legionella pneumophila* and *Mycoplasma* spp., if psittacosis is suspected, treatment should be commenced with a macrolide antibiotic.

A 40-year-old man with HIV presents with fever, dry cough, weight loss and exertional dyspnoea.

C This is a presentation of *Pneumocystis carinii* infection, which is a common complication of HIV infection (AIDS-defining illness). It may also occur as an opportunistic infection in other immunocompromised patients such as those receiving immunosuppressive drugs and cancer chemotherapy.

A 75-year-old man presents with headache, dry cough, anaemia and a skin rash. Blood tests detect cold agglutinins.

H Mycoplasma infection is the most common atypical cause of community-acquired pneumonia. Cases usually occur during an epidemic, which may give the clue to diagnosis. A characteristic feature is the autoimmune haemolytic anaemia caused by the presence of cold agglutinins. Other extrapulmonary features include erythema multiforme, myopericarditis and meningoencephalitis. Diagnosis is often made in retrospect via detection of a rising antibody titre. If mycoplasma infection is suspected on clinical grounds, a macrolide should be commenced empirically.

A 25-year-old air-conditioning technician, who suffered from flu-like symptoms a week ago, has developed a dry cough. His chest radiograph shows multilobar shadowing. Blood tests show hyponatraemia and lymphopenia. Urinalysis reveals haematuria.

A *Legionella pneumophila* is a rare cause of atypical community pneumonia. Cases may occur sporadically, although outbreaks associated with infected air-conditioning systems are well recognized. The patient often complains of a preceding flu-like illness before frank lower respiratory symptoms, e.g. dry cough and dyspnoea. Other features such as hyponatraemia and lymphopenia may assist in diagnosis, which can be performed rapidly by testing for the presence of legionella antigen in the urine (high sensitivity and specificity). Simple prevention measures such as adequate chlorination of the water supply are important to prevent outbreaks.

13 Haemoptysis

Answers: I G E A K

A 65-year-old smoker presents with shortness of breath, gallop rhythm and production of pink frothy sputum.

I This is the presentation of pulmonary oedema secondary to left ventricular failure as evidenced by the other cardiac signs, e.g. increased JVP, gallop rhythm. In this patient the most likely cause is ischaemic heart disease and there should be a high index of suspicion of an acute underlying ischaemic event, e.g. myocardial infarction.

A 24-year-old man initially complaining of cough and intermittent haemoptysis presents a few weeks later with haematuria. Biopsy confirms a crescentic glomerulonephritis. Renal biopsy shows linear pattern deposition on immunofluorescence.

G   This patient has presented with a pulmonary renal syndrome. Differential diagnosis includes Wegener's granulomatosis, microscopic polyangiitis and Goodpasture's disease (GD). Serology may assist in diagnosis in that Wegener's granulomatosis is associated with cANCA (cytoplasmic anti-neutrophil cytoplasmic antibody) (PR3) and anti-glomerular basement membrane (GBM) antibodies of the IgG type can be found in GD. The definitive diagnosis is made on renal biopsy where GD shows a classic linear staining on direct immunofluorescence. Renal biopsy also allows an assessment of the severity of the renal lesion.
GD is a condition resulting from the presence of anti-GBM antibodies. It is believed that the binding of these antibodies to the kidney glomerular membrane and lung alveolar membrane mediates a type II hypersensitivity reaction, which is responsible for the pathology in those organs. There is a strong association with HLA-DR2. The disease is said to occur more frequently in smokers and those exposed to the fumes of hydrocarbon solvents. Sufferers should avoid smoking, which can aggravate respiratory symptoms and increase the likelihood of lung haemorrhage. Treatment for this condition is immunosuppressive, e.g. corticosteroids, but plasmapheresis to remove the anti-GBM antibodies is also successful.

A 34-year-old woman originally complaining of nasal obstruction develops cough, haemoptysis and pleuritic chest pain. Her chest radiograph shows multiple nodular masses.

E   Wegener's granulomatosis is a small artery vasculitis (PR3 ANCA positive), which is characterized by lesions involving the upper respiratory tract, lungs and kidneys. Look out for eye signs that are present in up to 50 per cent, e.g. scleritis, uveitis, retinitis. However, the vasculitis and granuloma deposition can affect any organ and so less common associated symptoms and signs are legion. Treatment options include the use of immunosuppressive medications, e.g. high-dose corticosteroids with cyclophosphamide.

A 22-year-old man presents with fever, nightsweats, weight loss and cough productive of cupfuls of blood. Ziehl–Neelsen stain is positive for acid-fast bacilli (AFB).

A   The symptoms are suggestive of TB but the diagnosis is clinched by the presence of AFBs with Ziehl–Neelsen staining. Although the lung is the most commonly affected organ in TB, infection may present in other sites, e.g. urinary tract, bone, central nervous system (CNS). Miliary TB is the term used to describe widespread TB through haematological dissemination. It carries a poor prognosis.

A 35-year-old businessman returns from a trip abroad and collapses at the airport with haemoptysis and pleuritic chest pain. He has a sinus tachycardia and his ECG shows right axis deviation.

K   This is a classic history of pulmonary embolus (PE), although in many cases not all these features may be present. Diagnosis relies on a high index of clinical suspicion together with tests such as ventilation–perfusion scanning and pulmonary angiography (now commonly performed using spiral computed tomography). Other risk factors for PE include previous thromboembolic events, oral contraceptive pill, surgery (especially pelvic surgery), immobility and inherited thrombophilias.

14 Chest radiograph pathology

Answers: J M C F A

Multiple bilateral nodules between 0.5 and 5 cm in a former miner with rheumatoid arthritis.

J   Caplan's syndrome is a pulmonary manifestation of rheumatoid arthritis (RA) which is characterized by the presence of pulmonary nodules. It typically occurs in patients with RA who are exposed to coal dust, although the granulomas can also appear in workers exposed to other dusts, e.g. silicosis and asbestos. Symptoms include cough, shortness of breath and haemoptysis.
RA has several other respiratory manifestations/associations including fibrosing alveolitis, pleural effusions and, very rarely, obliterative bronchiolitis. RA can also affect the cricoarytenoid joints leading to upper respiratory tract obstruction.

Kerley B lines, bat-wing shadowing, prominent upper lobe vessels, cardiomegaly.

M   These findings are suggestive of acute left ventricular failure leading to pulmonary oedema. Kerley B lines are often difficult to see in real life. Although right ventricular failure may present with cardiomegaly, pulmonary oedema does not occur.

Trachea deviated to right, horizontal fissure and right hilum displaced upwards.

C   These chest radiograph findings are characteristic of right upper lobe collapse. Try to find the horizontal fissure because its position is a good clue to the presence of volume loss. The horizontal fissure on the right lung should run from the middle of the right hilum and can be traced to the level of the sixth rib in the axillary line. In right upper lobe collapse, the horizontal fissure will be elevated.

Chest radiograph findings of a left upper lobe collapse are somewhat different. There is no left middle lobe and hence no horizontal fissure. The upper lobe is anterior to a greater proportion of the lower lobe. Hence, left upper lobe collapse can give rise to a hazy white appearance over a large part of the left lung field. This should not be confused with a pleural effusion because in collapse there will be tracheal deviation to the side of the lesion, elevation of the hilum and preservation of the costophrenic angle.

Numerous calcified nodules sized less than 5 mm located predominantly in the lower zones of the lungs.

F   Multiple, small, calcified nodules may occur after varicella pneumonitis. Other causes of numerous calcified nodules include TB, histoplasmosis and chronic renal failure.

Double shadow right heart border, prominent left atrial appendage, left main bronchus elevation.

A   Advanced mitral stenosis is associated with characteristic findings caused by left atrial enlargement. These include elevation of the left main bronchus, widening of the carina, double right heart border and a prominent left atrial appendage. Calcification of the mitral valve may also be seen, as may pulmonary oedema. Left ventricular enlargement is not a feature despite the presence of pulmonary oedema.

15 Chest radiograph pathology

Answers: K C E F G

A 28-year-old African–Caribbean man presents with dry cough and progressive shortness of breath. His chest radiograph shows bilateral hilar lymphadenopathy.

K   This constellation of symptoms and radiological findings is highly suggestive of sarcoidosis which is more common in black patients. Other causes of bilateral hilar lymphadenopathy include TB, malignancy (although symmetrical lymphadenopathy is rare), organic dust diseases and extrinsic allergic alveolitis.

The chest radiograph of a 13-year-old boy with cystic fibrosis has tramline and ring shadows.

C   Ring shadows and tramlining are a characteristic radiological finding in bronchiectasis, which is a common early complication of cystic fibrosis. Patients present with a cough productive of large amounts of purulent sputum and there can be haemoptysis. On examination the patient may be clubbed with coarse inspiratory crackles that can be heard over the infected areas of lung.

Other causes of bronchiectasis include Kartagener's syndrome, pertussis and bronchial obstruction.

A 65-year-old dockyard worker presents with weight loss and shortness of breath. He is clubbed and cachectic. His chest radiograph shows pleural calcification and a lobulated pleural mass.

E   Mesothelioma is a consequence of previous asbestos exposure. The chest radiograph classically shows a mass with a lobulated margin. Pleural calcification suggests possible previous exposure to asbestos but, in the absence of other features, it is benign.

A 40-year-old woman presents with gross clubbing and progressive shortness of breath. Examination reveals fine end-inspiratory crackles. Her chest radiograph shows a ground-glass appearance of the lung.

F   Combination of shortness of breath, clubbing and fine end-inspiratory crackles suggests cryptogenic fibrosing alveolitis, which usually has an onset during middle age. Chest radiograph findings include ground-glass shadowing. As the disease progresses, a 'honeycomb' lung may develop. Fibrosing alveolitis is associated with rheumatoid arthritis, systemic sclerosis and ulcerative colitis. In these cases it is not referred to as cryptogenic.

A 65-year-old smoker presents with shortness of breath. On the chest radiograph, eight ribs can be seen anteriorly above the diaphragm on each side of the chest in the mid-clavicular line.

G   It is usual to see no more than six ribs anteriorly above the diaphragm in the mid-clavicular line, in a posteroanterior chest radiograph taken at full inspiration. The presence of more visible ribs suggests hyperexpansion which may occur in COPD.

16 Treatment of asthma and COPD

Answers: M K C B H

A 7-year-old girl with slight wheeze and shortness of breath despite inhaled salbutamol.

M N   This patient's symptoms may respond to inhaled salbutamol if it can be delivered effectively to the lungs. Use of a spacer improves delivery in children and patients with poor inhaler technique. In young patients, it is particularly important to optimize bronchodilator therapy as early initiation of corticosteroids may lead to growth retardation.

A 22-year-old student with mild asthma that needs treatment for occasional early morning wheeze.

K   This is step 1 of the British Thoracic Society (BTS) 2003 guidelines for
         the management of asthma.

         **A 17-year-old student complains that he has to use his salbutamol
         inhaler regularly to control wheezing.**

C   In patients who require frequent doses of inhaled bronchodilators to
         control symptoms regular inhaled corticosteroids should be used.
         This is a part of step 2 of the BTS 2003 guidelines for the management of
         asthma in adults. Step 2 refers to regular preventer therapy and involves
         the daily use of inhaled steroid at a dosage appropriate to the severity of
         disease.

         **A 32-year-old patient taking maximum dose-inhaled therapy and
         slow-release theophylline shows persistently inadequate control of
         symptoms.**

B   Although oral glucocorticoids should be avoided where possible because
         of long-term adverse effects, all other therapeutic opportunities have
         been exhausted in this patient.
         The use of oral steroids is a part of step 5 of the BTS 2003 guidelines for
         the management of asthma. A patient with such poorly controllable
         asthma should be under specialist care.

         **A 25-year-old woman requires add-on therapy because inhaled
         beclomethasone and salbutamol do not adequately combat her
         symptoms.**

H   Under the BTS 2003 guidelines there are two options for escalation of
         therapy for patients not adequately controlled with a regular bronchodilator
         inhaler and low-dose inhaled corticosteroids. Either a long action β
         agonist can be added, as is the case in this patient, or the dose of inhaled
         steroid can be increased. This is step 3 of the BTS 2003 guidelines.*

17 Emergency management: respiratory distress

Answers: D K L H C

         **A 65-year-old man with long-standing COPD presents with severe
         shortness of breath. He has been treated with oxygen and nebulized
         bronchodilators. An hour later: Pao_2 6.0 kPa (on max. O_2), $Paco_2$
         16.0 kPa, pH 7.2.**

D   This patient has a severe exacerbation of COPD and consequent type II
         respiratory failure that has responded poorly to medical therapy.
         Conventional management would involve formal intubation, ventilation
         and transfer to an intensive care unit (ICU). The use of non-invasive

* British Thoracic Society (2003) Guidelines for the Management of Asthma. *Thorax* 2003; 58 (suppl I).

intermittent positive pressure ventilation (NIPPV) in such patients has been associated with a reduction in the number of patients requiring formal intubation. This is advantageous because anaesthesia and intubation can be very difficult in a patient with respiratory failure. NIPPV should be tried unless the patient is in extremis. Successful NIPPV requires a conscious and cooperative patient.

A 17-year-old woman presents with wheeze and marked perioral swelling: Pao_2 7.0 kPa (on 28 per cent O_2), $Paco_2$ 4.1 kPa.

K   This is a classic presentation of acute anaphylaxis, e.g. a type I IgE-mediated hypersensitivity reaction. The symptoms and signs include rash, oedema, tachycardia, hypotension and wheeze. Laryngeal oedema giving rise to upper airway obstruction is particularly worrying because it may impede endotracheal intubation.

Initial treatment of choice is 0.5 ml epinephrine (adrenaline) 1:1000 solution (500 μg) delivered intramuscularly which can be repeated in the absence of clinical improvement or if deterioration occurs. Intravenous epinephrine is dangerous and should be given slowly only in a dilution of at least 1 in 10 000 in an immediately life-threatening situation, e.g. frank cardiac arrest.

A 14 year old with asthma presents with an acute severe asthma attack: Pao_2 10.0 kPa (on 28 per cent O_2), $Paco_2$ 8.0 kPa

L   The British Thoracic Society suggests that features of a severe asthma attack include peak expiratory flow rate (PEFR) <50 per cent predicted/best, respiration rate ≥25 breaths/min, pulse ≥110 beats/min and inability to complete a sentence with one breath.

Markers of a life-threatening attack include a PEFR < 33 per cent of predicted/best, silent chest, cyanosis, poor respiratory effort, bradycardia, arrhythmia, hypotension, exhaustion, confusion, Pao_2 < 8 kPa, acidosis with pH < 7.35, high $Paco_2$. Intubation and transfer to the ICU must be considered if the patient is not responding to drug therapy.

This patient is both hypoxic and retaining CO_2. This is a poor prognostic sign because people with acute asthma usually have a low CO_2. The presence of a high CO_2 is associated with imminent respiratory collapse. Despite elevated CO_2, 100 per cent O_2 should be given because, in this patient, there is no risk of respiratory depression resulting from a hypoxic ventilatory drive. Between attacks the patient's CO_2 should be within the normal range. It is a common mistake to restrict oxygen to patients with asthma and a high CO_2.

A 28-year-old man involved in a road traffic accident presents with severe respiratory distress. Examination reveals decreased expansion on the right side of the chest with mediastinal shift to the left.

H   Tension pneumothorax is a medical emergency and management should not be delayed by obtaining a chest radiograph. Air is being drawn into the pleural space with each inspiration but cannot escape during expiration.

The mediastinum is therefore shifted to the contralateral side. This prejudices both ventilation of the other lung and filling of the heart. In this scenario there is reduced expansion on the right side and mediastinal shift to the left, so decompression on the right side is indicated. A cannula must be inserted into the second intercostal space in the mid-clavicular line of the affected side until a functioning intercostal tube can be positioned.

A young man presents with an acute onset shortness of breath. Examination reveals decreased expansion on the right: Sao_2 95 per cent.

C   A chest radiograph is indicated here to confirm the diagnosis of pneumo-thorax and to assess the degree of collapse.
In healthy patients a small pneumothorax will often heal without further intervention. The patient should be observed for 6 hours and, if there is no increase in the size of the pneumothorax, may be discharged with early follow-up and repeated chest radiograph. Spontaneous pneumo-thoraces are relatively common in young adults (especially tall thin men) and older patients with emphysema. In patients with thoracic disease/large pneumothoraces, simple aspiration is recommended as first-line treatment. If this is unsuccessful, a chest drain will be required.

18 Management of COPD

Answers: A F L D H

A previously healthy 65-year-old smoker with early COPD complains of shortness of breath on exertion.

A   Stopping smoking, encouraging exercise and reducing obesity should all be encouraged. The use of inhaled bronchodilators is first-line pharmacological therapy for early COPD.

A 65-year-old woman with longstanding COPD presents with short-ness of breath and cough productive of coloured sputum.

F   This is the presentation for an infective exacerbation of COPD.

A 70-year-old man admitted with acute severe exacerbation of COPD does not respond to oxygen and nebulized bronchodilators.

L   If such a patient deteriorates on medical therapy, early use of NIPPV may improve outcome and avoid intubation.

A 65-year-old patient with advanced COPD treated with bronchodila-tors and steroids still feels breathless. His baseline Pao_2 is around 6.5 kPa.

D   Long-term oxygen therapy should be considered in clinically stable non-smokers with $Pao_2 < 7.3$ kPa. There is evidence to suggest that keeping the $Pao_2 > 8.0$ kPa for more than 15 h every day increases survival.

A 55-year-old patient with COPD requires regular add-on therapy after bronchodilators do not control symptoms.

H   Oral aminophylline taken before going to bed may be particularly helpful for patients complaining of symptoms in the early hours of the morning. Aminophylline should be used with care because it has a narrow therapeutic index. Signs of toxicity include nausea, vomiting and cardiac arrhythmias.

19 Treatment of respiratory infections

Answers: H E M K C

Standard therapy for community-acquired pneumococcal pneumonia not requiring hospital admission.

H   Oral erythromycin can be prescribed as an alternative if the patient is allergic to penicillin, or in combination with amoxicillin if an atypical organism is suspected.

A 35-year-old patient on the ward admitted to hospital 10 days ago presents with severe pneumonia.

E   This infection is hospital acquired and therefore the range of pathogens is likely to be different from those causing community-acquired pneumonia. Such pathogens include Gram-negative aerobes, e.g. *Pseudomonas* spp., and are often multiply antibiotic resistant. Third-generation cephalosporins, e.g. ceftazidime, have some anti-pseudomonal activity and can prove effective in these circumstances.

A 40-year-old builder presents with a severe community-acquired pneumonia. Atypical pathogens are suspected.

M   This is standard therapy for a severe community-acquired pneumonia. Rifampicin can be added empirically if there is a high clinical suspicion of legionella infection.

A 22-year-old human immunodeficiency virus (HIV)-positive individual on anti-retroviral therapy presents with *Pneumocystis carinii* pneumonia.

K   Treatment of choice is high-dose co-trimoxazole delivered intravenously for 2–3 weeks. Intravenous pentamidine may be used if co-trimoxazole is contraindicated or not tolerated. Corticosteroids are often used as an adjunct to treatment if there is hypoxaemia.

A 19-year-old man contracts pneumonia with symptoms of headache, fever and dry cough. Serology shows evidence of chlamydia infection.

C   Chlamydial pneumonia often presents with a biphasic illness: upper respiratory tract symptoms precede the pneumonia. Diagnosis is usually made retrospectively. Tetracycline is the treatment of choice.

REVISION BOXES

Respiratory medicine

Findings of respiratory examination are common in extended matching questions (EMQs) and can be confusing. Box 1 summarizes some findings that are highly suggestive of particular diagnoses that are likely to be found in the options.

Box 1 On respiratory examination

Findings	Diagnosis
• Hyperexpanded chest	COPD
	Chronic asthma
• Postural flapping tremor	Acute CO_2 retention
• Stony dull percussion	Pleural effusion
• Fine crepitations	Pulmonary oedema
	Pulmonary fibrosis
• Pleuritic chest pain	Pulmonary embolism, pneumonia, pneumothorax
• Stridor	Upper airway obstruction, e.g. foreign body, croup

Be aware that clubbing can be associated with several respiratory conditions and this non-specific sign may be mentioned in EMQs (Box 2).

Box 2 The clubbed respiratory patient

- Bronchial carcinoma
- Bronchiectasis
- Lung abscess
- Empyema
- Cystic fibrosis
- Cryptogenic fibrosing alveolitis
- Mesothelioma
- TB
- NOT asthma, COPD

Being aware of distinctive chest radiograph changes is very useful when tackling EMQs. Box 3 summarizes some pathologies that should spring to mind when you see particular phrases in EMQs.

Box 3 Chest radiograph [14, 15]

Radiological change	Pathology
• Kerley B lines Bat-wing shadowing	Heart failure
• Tram-line shadowing	Bronchiectasis
• Miliary shadowing	Miliary TB
• Wedge-shaped infarct	Pulmonary embolus
• 'Ground-glass' appearance	Fibrosis
'Honeycomb' appearance	Fibrosis (late)
• Pleural mass with lobulated margin	Mesothelioma

Box 4 summarizes some details to look out for in an EMQ which suggest a particular respiratory condition.

Box 4 Respiratory conditions

Factor indicating diagnosis	Condition
• Early-onset emphysema plus liver disease	α_1-Antitrypsin deficiency [57]
Fever, cough, shortness of breath hours after exposure to antigen (usually farmer after hay exposure) Positive serum precipitins	Extrinsic allergic alveolitis [11]
• Asymptomatic with bilateral hilar lymphadenopathy (BHL)/progressive shortness of breath/dry cough Non-pulmonary manifestations, e.g. erythema nodosum ↑ serum ACE (angiotensin-converting enzyme) or hypercalcaemia may be mentioned	Sarcoidosis [5, 15]
• History of recurrent chest infections, failure to thrive May mention steatorrhoea (pancreatic insufficiency) Positive sweat test (sodium, chloride >60 mmol/l)	Cystic fibrosis [11, 15, 74]
• Progressive dyspnoea and cyanosis Gross clubbing, fine end-inspiratory crackles Chest radiograph: ground-glass → honeycomb lung	Fibrosing alveolitis [15]

continued overleaf

continued

• Non-specific, e.g. fever, nightsweats, anorexia, haemoptysis Ziehl–Neelsen staining shows acid-fast bacilli (AFBs)	TB [13, 97]
• Swinging fever, copious foul-smelling sputum Usually patient has persistent, worsening pneumonia	Lung abscess

An EMQ may require you to identify the most likely infecting organism in a patient with pneumonia (Box 5).

Box 5 Causative agents in patients with pneumonia

Cause	Organism
• Positive cold agglutinins	Mycoplasma infection [12, 20]
• Occupation involving water systems	Legionella infection [12]
• Cavitating lung(s)	Staphylococcal/klebsiella infection
• Contact with birds	*Chlamydia psittaci* infection [12, 19]
• HIV +ve, bilateral hilar shadowing	*Pneumocystis carinii* pneumonia [12, 19, 87]

In examination EMQs certain drugs for respiratory conditions tend to be associated with particular side effects (Box 6).

Box 6 Side effects of drugs

Side effect	Drug
Peripheral neuropathy, hepatitis	Isoniazid
Orange-coloured tears/urine	Rifampicin
Deranged liver function tests (LFTs), hepatitis	
Retrobulbar neuritis (pain, loss of vision)	Ethambutol
Gout	Pyrazinamide
Tremor, tachycardia	Salbutamol
Candidiasis mouth/pharynx	Inhaled high-dose corticosteroid

SECTION 3: HAEMATOLOGY AND ONCOLOGY

QUESTIONS

20 Causes of anaemia

A	autoimmune haemolytic anaemia	G	thalassaemia
B	spherocytosis	H	iron deficiency anaemia
C	pyruvate kinase deficiency	I	sickle-cell anaemia
D	aplastic anaemia	J	folate deficiency
E	thalassaemia minor	K	sideroblastic anaemia
F	glucose-6-phosphate dehydrogenase deficiency	L	pernicious anaemia

For each clinical scenario below, give the most likely cause for the clinical findings. Each option may be used only once.

1   A 23-year-old man presents with recurrent nose-bleeds and infection after a course of chemotherapy.

2   A 24-year-old Cypriot man presents with a worsening anaemia and jaundice. A blood film taken several weeks after the incident shows the presence of Heinz bodies.

3   A 50-year-old man presents with tiredness, dyspnoea and paraesthesia. On examination he showed extensor plantars, brisk knee jerks and absent ankle jerks. His blood film shows macrocytic anaemia.

4   A 23-year-old woman on trimethoprim for recurrent urinary tract infections (UTIs) presents with a macrocytic anaemia.

5   A 25-year-old woman with systemic lupus erythematosus (SLE) presents with an acute anaemia. She was successfully treated with steroids. Direct Coombs' test was strongly positive; direct antiglobulin test was positive with IgG alone.

Answers: see page 60.

21 Anaemia

A	sickle-cell disease	G	sideroblastic anaemia
B	pyruvate kinase deficiency	H	thalassaemia major
C	haemophilia A	I	aplastic anaemia
D	hereditary spherocytosis	J	iron deficiency anaemia
E	autoimmune haemolytic	K	thalassaemia minor
	anaemia	L	anaemia of chronic disease
F	vitamin B_{12} deficiency anaemia		

For each clinical scenario below, give the most likely cause for the clinical findings. Each option may be used only once.

1 A 70-year-old woman with rheumatoid arthritis presents with a normocytic normochromic anaemia: Hb 10.1 g/dl. Haematinics normal, direct Coombs' test negative.

2 A 24-year-old woman with anaemia and splenomegaly is referred to the haematologist. Her direct Coombs' test is negative. Her blood film shows the presence of reticulocytes and spherocytes.

3 A 17-year-old tourist from the West Indies presents with pain in his abdomen and hands. He is pyrexial and anaemic.

4 Full blood count of a 65-year-old woman taking ibuprofen for her osteoarthritic knee pain for a number of years shows a microcytic anaemia.

5 Full blood count of a 45-year-old man treated for gastric carcinoma with total gastrectomy reveals a macrocytic anaemia.

Answers: see page 61.

22 The peripheral blood film

A	vitamin B_{12} deficiency anaemia	G	hyposplenism
B	thalassaemia β	H	hypersplenism
C	hypothyroidism	I	bone marrow failure
D	haemophilia B	J	iron deficiency anaemia
E	uraemia	K	anaemia of chronic disease
F	sickle-cell anaemia	L	none of the above

For each finding from a peripheral blood film below, suggest the most likely cause for the result observed. Each option may be used only once.

1 Presence of Burr cells in a patient being treated in the intensive care unit (ICU) with multiple organ failure.

2 Howell–Jolly bodies in a patient with coeliac disease.

3 Neutrophil hypersegmentation in a patient with paraesthesia in the fingers and toes.

4 Microcytic hypochromic film in a 24-year-old woman presenting with lethargy.

5 Film of a 3-month-old baby boy shows a hypochromic microcytic anaemia with target cells and nucleated red blood cells. There are markedly high HbF levels.

Answers: see page 63.

23 Haematological diseases

A	myeloma	G	acute lymphoblastic leukaemia
B	Hodgkin's lymphoma	H	Burkitt's lymphoma
C	polycythaemia rubra vera	I	paroxysmal nocturnal haemo-
D	amyloidosis		globinuria
E	chronic lymphocytic leukaemia	J	essential thrombocythaemia
F	Waldenström's macroglobuli-	K	chronic myeloid leukaemia
	naemia	L	antiphospholipid syndrome

For each clinical scenario below, give the most likely cause for the clinical findings. Each option may be used only once.

1 A 25-year-old man presents with enlarged painless lymph nodes in the neck. His peripheral blood film shows Reed–Sternberg cells.

2 A 45-year-old man presents with fever, weight loss, tiredness and gout. On examination there is splenomegaly. White blood cell count is $112 \times 10^9/l$. The Philadelphia chromosome is detected.

3 A 70-year-old woman complains of weight loss, headache, blurry vision, lethargy and haematuria. Positive findings on examination include cervical lymphadenopathy, splenomegaly and numerous retinal haemorrhages. Bone marrow biopsy shows lymphoplasmacytoid cell infiltrate.

4 A 27-year-old man presents with haemolytic anaemia after surgery. He reports a history of recurrent abdominal pains. The Ham's test is positive.

5 A 60-year-old man presents with headaches, blurred vision and itching over the whole body (the last after a hot bath). Positive findings on examination include plethoric facies and moderate splenomegaly. Haematocrit: 65 per cent.

Answers: see page 64.

24 Cancer care

A   hyoscine butylbromide
B   hyoscine, midazolam
C   paracetamol
D   haloperidol, midazolam
E   ondansetron
F   dexamethasone

G   metoclopramide, phenytoin, hyoscine
H   metoclopramide
I   morphine
J   ibuprofen
K   amitriptyline
L   co-dydramol

For each clinical scenario below, suggest the most appropriate management. Each option may be used only once.

1   A 65-year-old lung cancer patient with brain metastases is suffering from severe headache. He has papilloedema in both eyes.

2   A 60-year-old man with metastatic colorectal carcinoma is suffering from severe pain.

3   A 50-year-old man requires first-line pain relief for bony metastases.

4   A 55-year-old patient with metastatic cancer from an unknown primary requires medication to treat convulsions, vomiting and terminal restlessness.

5   A 30-year-old man undergoing chemotherapy for teratoma is suffering from severe vomiting shortly after receiving the drug.

Answers: see page 65.

25 Tumour markers

A PSA (prostate-specific antigen)
B ADH
C calcitonin
D β–hCG (β–human chorionic gonadotrophin)
E CA 19–9
F CA 15–3

G AFP (α–fetoprotein)
H ANP
I 5 HIAA
J urinary catecholamines
K PTH
L CEA (carcinoembryonic antigen)

For each of the presentations of cancer below, suggest the tumour marker that is most likely to be elevated.

1 A 60-year-old man presents with poor stream, weight loss and back pain. Digital rectal examination reveals a hard irregular prostate gland.

2 A 65-year-old woman with weight loss and painless jaundice. There is evidence of thrombophlebitis migrans and computed tomography (CT) shows a mass in the pancreatic head.

3 A 70-year-old man presenting with a suspected recurrence of colorectal carcinoma.

4 A 68-year-old person with chronic alcohol problems and hepatocellular carcinoma.

5 A 34-year-old man is referred to radiotherapy with seminoma.

Answers: see page 66.

26 Risk factors for malignancy

A	nasopharyngeal carcinoma	H	prostatic carcinoma
B	ovarian carcinoma	G	gastrointestinal lymphoma
C	gastric carcinoma	I	bronchial carcinoma
D	oesophageal carcinoma	J	cervical carcinoma
E	breast carcinoma	K	bladder carcinoma
F	colorectal carcinoma		

Choose the malignancy that is most strongly associated with the risk factor below. Each option may be used only once.

1 Previous exposure to aniline dyes.

2 Epstein–Barr virus infection in a native African.

3 Coeliac disease.

4 Pernicious anaemia.

5 Unprotected sexual intercourse with several sexual partners.

Answers: see page 67.

27 Adverse effects of chemotherapy

A paclitaxel
B folic acid
C prednisolone
D mesna
E bleomycin
F dihydrotestosterone
G flutamide

H trimethoprim
I erythromycin
J doxorubicin
K chlorambucil
L 5-fluorouracil
M cyclophosphamide
N tamoxifen

For each scenario, choose the drug most likely to be responsible for the adverse effects encountered. Each option may be used only once.

1 A 66-year-old woman treated with an alkylating agent for myeloma presents with severe haematuria.

2 A 34-year-old woman treated with a microtubular inhibitor for carcinoma of the breast develops a peripheral neuropathy.

3 A young man treated with an antibiotic for acute leukaemia develops arrhythmias and heart block shortly after the administration of chemotherapy.

4 A patient treated with an antibiotic for lung cancer develops pulmonary fibrosis.

5 A 55-year-old man on treatment for prostate cancer complains of gynaecomastia.

Answers: see page 67.

ANSWERS

20 Causes of anaemia

Answers: D F L J A

> A 23-year-old man presents with recurrent nose-bleeds and infection after a course of chemotherapy.

D   Aplastic anaemia is a presentation of pancytopenia with hypoplastic marrow. Aplastic anaemia can be either primary or secondary. The most common cause of primary aplastic anaemia is idiopathic acquired aplastic anaemia. Congenital causes of primary aplastic anaemia are very rare, e.g. Fanconi's anaemia. Secondary causes of aplastic anaemia include infection (especially viral, e.g. hepatitis, measles, parvovirus B19) and drugs. Cytotoxic drugs such as busulphan and doxorubicin are well-recognized causes of secondary aplastic anaemia via a type A (dose-related) response. Non-cytotoxic drugs such as chloramphenicol and gold have also been reported to cause aplasia via a type B (not dose-related) response. Rarely, pregnancy is associated with a secondary aplastic anaemia.

> A 24-year-old Cypriot man presents with a worsening anaemia and jaundice. A blood film taken several weeks after the incident shows the presence of Heinz bodies.

F   Glucose-6-phosphate dehydrogenase (G6PDH) deficiency is the most common red blood cell enzyme defect and is more common in patients of Mediterranean origin. Individuals with this condition are susceptible to oxidative crises precipitated by fava beans and drugs such as ciprofloxacin and sulphonamides. G6PDH plays an important role in the hexose monophosphate shunt which provides NADPH (reduced nicotinamide adenine dinucleotide phosphate – the reducing agent). NADPH is used to regenerate glutathione. In the absence of glutathione, red blood cells are exposed to oxidative stress. Heinz bodies represent oxidized haemoglobin.

> A 50-year-old man presents with tiredness, dyspnoea and paraesthesia. On examination he showed extensor plantars, brisk knee jerks and absent ankle jerks. His blood film shows macrocytic anaemia.

L   Pernicious anaemia is the most common cause of vitamin B_{12} deficiency. This is an autoimmune condition characterized by atrophy of the gastric mucosa with subsequent failure of intrinsic factor production. Intrinsic factor is required for vitamin B_{12} absorption. Other causes of vitamin B_{12} deficiency are terminal ileum disease, gastrectomy and low dietary intake (e.g. vegans).

It is important to establish the cause of the vitamin B_{12} deficiency because this affects management. Dietary deficiency can be treated with oral vitamin B_{12} whereas parenteral vitamin B_{12} (e.g. intramuscular hydroxocobalamin) is required for pernicious anaemia.

A 23-year-old woman on trimethoprim for recurrent urinary tract infections (UTIs) presents with a macrocytic anaemia.

J   Causes of macrocytosis include vitamin B_{12}/folate deficiency, alcohol, liver disease, hypothyroidism and myelodysplasia. Trimethoprim is a bacterial dihydrofolate reductase inhibitor, but with prolonged therapy it may act as a human dihydrofolate reductase inhibitor. It is avoided in pregnancy because the interference with folate metabolism could prove teratogenic.

Bone marrow biopsy is indicated if the cause of the macrocytosis is not established with blood tests.

A 25-year-old woman with SLE presents with an acute anaemia. She was successfully treated with steroids. A direct Coombs' test was strongly positive; direct antiglobulin test was positive with IgG alone.

A   There are many causes of anaemia in a patient with SLE, including iron deficiency anaemia secondary to non-steroidal anti-inflammatory drug (NSAID) use and bone marrow suppression secondary to immunosuppressive drugs, e.g. cyclophosphamide/azathioprine. Autoimmune haemolytic anaemia (AHA) is the cause of anaemia in this patient. A direct Coombs' test demonstrates and confirms the presence of antibody binding to red blood cells.

Other causes of secondary AHA include lymphoma, infections (e.g. Epstein–Barr virus [EBV], *Mycoplasma* spp.), carcinoma and other autoimmune conditions.

Some drugs may also cause an immune haemolysis, e.g. methyldopa treatment can induce the formation of red cell autoantibodies.

21 Anaemia

Answers: L D A J F

A 70-year-old woman with rheumatoid arthritis presents with a normocytic normochromic anaemia: Hb 10.1 g/dl. Haematinics normal, direct Coombs' test negative.

L   Anaemia of chronic disease is associated with many chronic inflammatory diseases and malignancy. This anaemia is mild and normocytic, so it is incorrect to attribute an anaemia with Hb < 8 g/dl to chronic disease. All other causes for the anaemia must be ruled out before making the diagnosis of anaemia of chronic disease.

A 24-year-old woman with anaemia and splenomegaly is referred to the haematologist. Her direct Coombs' test is negative. Her blood film shows the presence of reticulocytes and spherocytes.

D   Hereditary spherocytosis is a genetic defect in the red cell membrane structure. Most cases are inherited in an autosomal dominant fashion but the patient can also present without family history as a result of spontaneous mutation. Patients may present with jaundice at birth but can also remain asymptomatic for many years. The direct Coombs' test is negative in hereditary spherocytosis. This is an important test because spherocytes are also commonly found in autoimmune haemolytic anaemia.

Treatment of choice is splenectomy because the spleen is the site of spherocyte removal.

A 17-year-old tourist from the West Indies presents with pain in his abdomen and hands. He is pyrexial and anaemic.

A   Sickle-cell anaemia results from an amino acid substitution in the gene coding for the β chain of Hb, giving rise to altered Hb known as HbS. HbS polymerizes when deoxygenated, producing characteristically sickle-shaped cells. This results in both a haemolytic anaemia and occlusion of small blood vessels.

Several sickle-cell crises are recognized:

(i)   Infarctive crises give rise to the painful hand and foot syndrome, avascular necrosis of the femoral head, splenic infarction and priapism. A patient with hepatosplenomegaly may be suffering from a sequestration crisis where sickle cells have been trapped in the liver and spleen.

(ii)   Haemolytic crisis resulting in jaundice may be precipitated by an infection, drug, etc.

(iii)   Aplastic crises may occur secondary to infection (usually by parvovirus).

Full blood count of a 65-year-old woman taking ibuprofen for her osteoarthritic knee pain for a number of years shows a microcytic anaemia.

J   Iron deficiency anaemia classically causes a microcytosis. The most likely cause in this case is loss from the gastrointestinal tract as a result of chronic NSAID use.

Full blood count of a 45-year-old man treated for gastric carcinoma with total gastrectomy reveals a macrocytic anaemia.

F   Intrinsic factor secreted by the stomach is required for vitamin B_{12} absorption. The Schilling test can be used to determine whether low serum vitamin B_{12} is the result of malabsorption from the terminal ileum or lack of intrinsic factor secreted by the stomach.

22 The peripheral blood film

Answers: E G A J B

> Presence of Burr cells in a patient being treated in the ICU with multiple organ failure.

E Burr cells indicate uraemia.

> Howell–Jolly bodies in a patient with coeliac disease.

G Howell–Jolly bodies are found in hyposplenism.

> Neutrophil hypersegmentation in a patient with paraesthesia in the fingers and toes.

A Vitamin B_{12} deficiency is a recognized cause of megaloblastic anaemia and, if left untreated, can lead to a polyneuropathy affecting the peripheral nerves. There is early loss of vibration sense and proprioception because the posterior columns are affected first.
Other changes in megaloblastic anaemia include chromatin deficiency, premature haemoglobinization and the presence of giant metamyelocytes.

> Microcytic hypochromic film in a 24-year-old woman presenting with lethargy.

J Target cells are a feature of iron deficiency anaemia. Koilonychia (brittle spoon-shaped nails) are found in severe disease. Other rare signs include angular cheilosis and oesophageal web. The presence of an iron deficiency anaemia plus oesophageal web is known as the Plummer–Vinson/Paterson–Brown–Kelly syndrome.

> Film of a 3-month-old baby boy shows a hypochromic microcytic anaemia with target cells and nucleated red blood cells. There are markedly high HbF levels.

B In β-thalassaemia there is defective synthesis of β chains with a severity that depends on the inheritance of the defect. A patient with thalassaemia minor is an asymptomatic heterozygous carrier. The thalassaemia major patient is homozygous and usually presents in the first year of life with a severe anaemia and failure to thrive. The symptoms of anaemia start at this point because this is the period when γ chain production is switched off and β chains fail to form in adequate numbers.
Blood transfusions are required to keep the Hb > 9–10 g/dl. Iron chelators are required to protect the major organs from transfusion-mediated iron overload. Ascorbic acid (vitamin C) can also be used to increase urinary excretion of iron. The patient requires long-term folic acid supplements caused by the extreme demand associated with bone marrow hyperplasia.

23 Haematological diseases

Answers: B K F I C

> A 25-year-old man presents with enlarged painless lymph nodes in the neck. His peripheral blood film shows Reed–Sternberg cells.

B   Reed–Sternberg cells are classically binucleate and pathognomonic of Hodgkin's lymphoma. The two large nuclei can give rise to an owl's eye appearance.

> A 45-year-old man presents with fever, weight loss, tiredness and gout. On examination there is splenomegaly. White blood cell count is $112 \times 10^9/l$. The Philadelphia chromosome is detected.

K   Chronic myeloid leukaemia (CML) is a myeloproliferative disorder characterized by uncontrolled proliferation of myeloid cells where the white cell count is often $>100 \times 10^9/l$. The highest incidence of CML is in middle age. Myeloproliferative and lymphoproliferative disorders can be associated with hyperuricaemia and thus gout caused by increased turnover of purines. The Philadelphia chromosome, a translocation between the long arm of chromosome 22 to chromosome 9, is seen in around 95 per cent patients. Treatment options include the use of interferon, hydroxyurea and allogeneic transplantation from a suitable donor.

> A 70-year-old woman complains of weight loss, headache, blurry vision, lethargy and haematuria. Positive findings on examination include cervical lymphadenopathy, splenomegaly and numerous retinal haemorrhages. Bone marrow biopsy shows lymphoplasmacytoid cell infiltrate.

F   Waldenström's macroglobulinaemia (WM) is a lymphoplasmacytoid lymphoma that usually affects older men. The clinical manifestations of the disease, e.g. hyperviscosity, result from the production of IgM paraprotein. Myeloma can also give signs of hyperviscosity, but splenomegaly and lymphadenopathy make WM more likely. Bone marrow biopsy shows the presence of lymphoplasmacytoid cells. There are usually very few plasma cells unlike myeloma, which shows a characteristic infiltrate of plasma cells.

> A 27-year-old man presents with haemolytic anaemia after surgery. He reports a history of recurrent abdominal pains. The Ham's test is positive.

I   Paroxysmal nocturnal haemoglobinuria (PNH) is an acquired defect where red cells are unusually sensitive to destruction by activated complement. Patients may present non-specifically with recurrent abdominal pains or with haemolytic anaemia. Venous thrombotic episodes are very common in patients with PNH. The condition acquired its name from the characteristic finding of dark-coloured urine when voiding at night or early in the morning.

In Ham's test, the cells from a PNH patient will lyse more readily in acid-
ified serum than normal red blood cells. Serum heated to around 56°C
will inactivate complement and thus haemolysis will not occur.
As a result of the high risk of venous thrombosis, long-term coagulation
may be necessary. Deficient haematopoeisis may also occur and PNH
may progress to aplastic anaemia in around 10–20 per cent individuals.

**A 60-year-old man presents with headaches, blurred vision and itch-
ing over the whole body (the last after a hot bath). Positive findings
on examination include plethoric facies and moderate splenomegaly.
Haematocrit: 65 per cent.**

C   Polycythaemia rubra vera (PRV) is a primary polycythaemia where there
is excessive proliferation of red blood cells caused by a clonal disorder of
pluripotent stem cells. The condition usually presents in late middle age –
elderly patients with signs of hyperviscosity, e.g. blurry vision (retinal
haemorrhages), headaches, bleeding, etc. Severe pruritus after a hot bath
is a commonly reported finding. The patient typically has plethoric facies
and may be cyanotic as a result of stagnation and deoxygenation of the
blood in peripheral vessels. Splenomegaly is very common in PRV, unlike
secondary polycythaemia. Blood tests show an elevated packed cell
volume. The white cell count is usually raised. A raised red cell mass can
be shown with ^{51}Cr studies.
The aim of treatment is to normalize the full blood count and prevent the
complications of thrombosis and haemorrhage. Venesection is the treatment of choice. Hydroxyurea chemotherapy can also be used to control
thrombocytosis.

24 Cancer care

Answers: F I J D E

**A 65-year-old lung cancer patient with brain metastases is suffering
from severe headache. He has papilloedema in both eyes.**

F   Dexamethasone is used in the short term to reduce the raised intracranial
pressure caused by cerebral oedema around metastases.

**A 60-year-old man with metastatic colorectal carcinoma is suffering
from severe pain.**

I   Severe pain from terminal malignancy often requires the use of strong
opioids. The most common adverse effect is constipation. If morphine is
being used regularly (e.g. in terminal care), a laxative should also be
prescribed to limit constipation.

A 50-year-old man requires first-line pain relief for bony metastases.

J   NSAIDs are a very effective first-line analgesic for bony metastases.

A 55-year-old patient with metastatic cancer from an unknown primary requires medication to treat convulsions, vomiting and terminal restlessness.

D   Midazolam is used to treat both convulsions and terminal restlessness.

A 30-year-old man undergoing chemotherapy for teratoma is suffering from severe vomiting shortly after receiving the drug.

E   Vomiting during cancer chemotherapy is common and can be classified as anticipatory, immediate or delayed. Anticipatory symptoms can be controlled with a benzodiazepine, e.g. diazepam. Corticosteroids, e.g. dexamethasone, can be used to treat delayed vomiting. Ondansetron is a serotonin $5HT_3$ antagonist that is used for immediate severe vomiting, particularly in those individuals receiving highly emetogenic chemotherapy.

25 Tumour markers

Answers: A E L G D

A 60-year-old man presents with poor stream, weight loss and back pain. Digital rectal examination reveals a hard irregular prostate gland.

A   This is a presentation of carcinoma of the prostate. The benefit of screening asymptomatic men with respect to increased later survival is unclear. PSA may also be raised in benign prostatic hypertrophy. It is always important to remember that a patient with carcinoma of the prostate may have a normal PSA. PSA levels increase with age and therefore the reference range for 'normal values' also changes.

A 65-year-old woman with weight loss and painless jaundice. There is evidence of thrombophlebitis migrans and computed tomography (CT) shows a mass in the pancreatic head.

E   CA 19-9 is usually raised in patients with pancreatic carcinoma (around 80 per cent). CEA can also be raised in pancreatic carcinoma but this is less common (around 40–50 per cent). The use of CA 19-9 is very limited diagnostically because it can be raised in other malignancies and benign processes, e.g. cirrhosis, cholangitis.

A 70-year-old man presenting with a suspected recurrence of colorectal carcinoma.

L   CEA can be used clinically to monitor response to treatment. As with most tumour markers, it is not specific enough to be of diagnostic value.

A 68-year-old person with chronic alcohol problems and hepatocellular carcinoma.

G   Hepatocellular carcinoma is associated with a raised AFP level. It is also raised in germ-cell tumours, hepatitis and pregnancy.

A 34-year-old man is referred to radiotherapy with seminoma.

D   β-hCG is also raised in choriocarcinoma. Unlike teratoma, AFP is not raised in seminoma.

26 Risk factors for malignancy

Answers: K A H C J

Previous exposure to aniline dyes.

K   Contact with aniline dyes is associated with bladder cancer.

Epstein–Barr virus infection in a native African.

A   Epstein–Barr virus infection is a risk factor for Burkitt's lymphoma, post-transplant lymphoma and HIV-associated lymphoma.

Coeliac disease.

H   There is an increased incidence of T-cell lymphoma and adenocarcinoma of the small bowel.

Pernicious anaemia.

C   Pernicious anaemia is associated with later gastric carcinoma.

Unprotected sexual intercourse with several sexual partners.

J   Transmission of human papilloma virus is believed to be relevant in the association of cervical cancer with unprotected sexual intercourse with many partners.

27 Adverse effects of chemotherapy

Answers: M A J E G

A 66-year-old woman treated with an alkylating agent for myeloma presents with severe haematuria.

M   Haemorrhagic cystitis is caused by toxic metabolites of cyclophosphamide, e.g. acrolein. Mesna is a uroprotective agent that can be given orally or by intravenous injection to react specifically with this metabolite in the urinary tract and prevent toxicity.

A 34-year-old woman treated with a microtubular inhibitor for carcinoma of the breast develops a peripheral neuropathy.

A   Microtubular inhibitors include the vinca alkaloids, e.g. vinblastine, vincristine, and the taxanes, e.g. paclitaxel, docetaxel. Tubulin is a protein that is essential for formation of the spindle that separates the chromosomes during mitosis.
Neurotoxicity occurs as a result of involvement of microtubules concerned with neuronal growth and axonal transport.

A young man treated with an antibiotic for acute leukaemia develops arrhythmias and heart block shortly after the administration of chemotherapy.

J   Doxorubicin, an anthracycline antibiotic, is widely used for the treatment of acute leukaemias, lymphomas and solid tumours. Cardiotoxicity is a well-recognized adverse effect and can be manifested as acute arrhythmias, developing shortly after drug administration or as chronic cardiomyopathy. The cumulative dose is usually limited to reduce risk of cardiomyopathy and consequent congestive heart failure.
Alopecia is a very common adverse effect of doxorubicin treatment and can be counteracted to some extent by scalp cooling.

A patient treated with an antibiotic for lung cancer develops pulmonary fibrosis.

E   Progressive pulmonary fibrosis is a dose-related adverse effect of bleomycin treatment.

A 55-year-old man on treatment for prostate cancer complains of gynaecomastia.

G   Hormonal treatment of advanced metastatic prostate cancer involves targeting the androgen dependence of those tumour cells. Gonadotrophin-releasing hormone analogues, e.g. goserelin, stimulate and then reduce pituitary follicle-stimulating hormone (FSH) and luteinizing hormone (LH) release. The initial rise in FSH/LH gives rise to a 'tumour flare', with progression of cancer and worsening of symptoms. Cyproterone acetate and flutamide are dihydrotestosterone receptor blockers used to treat the 'tumour flare' associated with treatment with gonadotrophin-releasing hormone analogues.

REVISION BOXES

Haematology and oncology

Results of the peripheral blood film are often a good clue to the answer in an EMQ (Box 1).

Box 1 On the peripheral blood film [22]

Film	Condition
Howell–Jolly bodies	Hyposplenism
Burr cells	Uraemia
Heinz bodies	Glucose-6-phosphate dehydrogenase deficiency
Reticulocytosis	Bleeding, haemolysis
Target cells	Liver disease, iron deficiency anaemia

The patient with anaemia is frequently found in EMQs. You should be aware of all the causes of a macrocytic, microcytic and normochromic anaemia because this will rapidly help you to eliminate options.

Box 2 summarizes some features of causes of anaemia that are common in EMQs.

Box 2 Anaemia [21]

Patient has macrocytic anaemia:

- With glossitis, peripheral neuropathy   Vitamin B_{12} deficiency
- And is on drugs, e.g. phenytoin,   Folate deficiency
  trimethoprim
- With dry, thin hair, slowly relaxing   Hypothyroidism
  reflexes
- Alcohol can cause a macrocytic anaemia
  and a macrocytosis without anaemia

Patient has microcytic anaemia:

- And menorrhagia   Iron deficiency anaemia
- And is on chronic NSAID (non-steroidal   Iron deficiency anaemia
  anti-inflammatory drug) treatment
- With an increased HbF   β-Thalassaemia

continued overleaf

continued

Normocytic anaemia:

Look out for anaemia of chronic disease (AOCD), e.g. malignancy, rheumatoid arthritis
Anaemia is mild, if Hb $<$ 8 g/dl it cannot be called AOCD
Endocrine dysfunction can give a normocytic anaemia

Haematological diseases:

Young black patient presenting with anaemia, jaundice: Hand and foot syndrome (painful infarcts) 'Sickle chest' (fever, pain, mimics pneumonia) Priapism leading to impotence Hepatosplenomegaly (sequestration crisis)	Sickle-cell anaemia [21]
• Patient of Mediterranean origin:	Glucose-6-phosphate dehydrogenase deficiency [20]
• Rapid anaemia, jaundice and Heinz bodies Precipitated by fava beans, sulphonamides	
• Skull bossing, maxillary hypertrophy, ↑ HbF	β-Thalassaemia [22]
• Bleeds excessively (e.g. into joints and muscle) ↓↓ factor VIII assay	Haemophilia A
• Dark urine in the morning Positive Ham's test	Paroxysmal nocturnal haemoglobinuria [23]

A presentation of malignancy is a common scenario in an EMQ and you should be able to recognize various classic presentations of malignancy and look for them immediately in the options given to you (Box 3).

Box 3 Presentation of malignancy

Presentation	Type of cancer
EMQ usually includes weight loss plus:	
• Anaemia, dysphagia	Oesophageal carcinoma
• Painless obstructive jaundice	Carcinoma head of pancreas
• Painless total haematuria	Bladder carcinoma
• Haemoptysis, smoking history	Bronchial carcinoma
• Change in bowel habit, per bleeding	Colorectal carcinoma
• Flushing, abdominal pain, diarrhoea, heart failure	Carcinoid syndrome
• Bladder outflow obstruction, bone pain (metastatic)	Carcinoma of the prostate

In an EMQ involving haematological malignancy as a possible option, it is particularly important to be aware of classic features on blood film/bone marrow biopsy (Box 4).

Box 4 Haematological malignancy

• Reed–Sternberg cells	Hodgkin's lymphoma [23]
• Auer rods	Acute myeloid leukaemia
• Middle age, ↑↑↑ WCC (white cell count), gout, Philadelphia chromosome	Chronic myeloid leukaemia
• Usually elderly patient Bone pain very common Look out for renal failure Hyperviscosity, e.g. retinal haemorrhages Monoclonal Ig band on electrophoresis Bone marrow biopsy: plasma cell infiltration	Myeloma [45, 82]

In exam EMQs certain drugs tend to be associated with particular side effects (Box 5).

Box 5 Adverse effects of chemotherapy [27]

Drug	Effect
Doxorubicin	Cardiotoxicity
Bleomycin, methotrexate, busulphan	Pulmonary fibrosis
Cyclophosphamide	Haemorrhagic cystitis
Vinca alkaloids, e.g. vincristine, platinum compounds, e.g. cisplatin, taxanes, e.g. paclitaxel	Peripheral neuropathy

SECTION 4: NEUROLOGY

QUESTIONS

28 Dizziness and vertigo

A   vertebrobasilar ischaemia
B   benign positional vertigo
C   vestibular schwannoma
D   lateral medullary syndrome
E   multiple sclerosis
F   Menière's disease
G   auditory eczema

H   acoustic neuroma
I   vestibular neuronitis
J   Ramsay Hunt syndrome
K   migraine
L   perilymph fistula
M   hyperventilation

For each clinical scenario below, give the most likely cause for the clinical findings. Each option may be used only once.

1   A 45-year-old woman presents with a left-sided facial palsy and vertigo. She has impaired hearing on her left side and a vesicular rash is noted around her external auditory meatus.

2   A 55-year-old man presents with a history of recurrent spontaneous attacks of vertigo, hearing loss and tinnitus. These attacks last up to 2 h and are sometimes associated with vomiting.

3   A 65-year-old woman presents with vertigo, vomiting and dysphagia. On examination there is a left-sided Horner's syndrome, and loss of pain and temperature on the right side of the face.

4   A 50-year-old man presents with vertigo when rolling over quickly in bed, getting out of bed and bending over. His hearing is normal.

5   A 20-year-old man presents with vertigo having suffered with symptoms of flu for several days.

Answers: see page 88.

29 Headache

A	tension headache	H	meningitis
B	migraine	I	sinusitis
C	amaurosis fugax	J	cluster headache
D	epilepsy	K	analgesic headache
E	subdural haematoma	L	giant cell arteritis
F	subarachnoid haemorrhage	M	episcleritis
G	encephalitis		

For each clinical scenario below, give the most likely cause for the clinical findings. Each option may be used only once.

1   A 40-year-old man complains of severe headache of sudden onset 4 h ago, likened to being kicked in the back of the head. He has vomited twice and is now feeling stiff in his neck.

2   A 40-year-old businesswoman complains of a headache that feels like a tight band around her head.

3   A 55-year-old woman presents with a headache that has lasted a few weeks. She gets pain in her jaw during meals and her scalp is tender on palpation.

4   A 30-year-old man complains of rapid-onset pain around his left eye every night for the last 2 weeks, associated with lid swelling, watery eye and flushing. He suffers from these bouts every 3 months.

5   A 24-year-old woman complains of a unilateral throbbing headache lasting 6 hours associated with vomiting and photophobia. She has had several episodes in the past.

Answers: see page 89.

30 Headache

A	cluster headache	H	migraine
B	uveitis	I	meningitis
C	scleritis	J	space-occupying lesion
D	acute glaucoma	K	migrainous neuralgia
E	subdural haematoma	L	trigeminal neuralgia
F	subarachnoid haemorrhage	M	febrile convulsion
G	benign intracranial hypertension		

For each clinical scenario below, give the most likely cause for the clinical findings. Each option may be used only once.

1   A 56-year-old woman complains of unilateral stabbing pain on the surface of her scalp and around her eye. The pain is precipitated by washing or touching the specific area.

2   A 28-year-old woman complains of headache and double vision which is worse when lying down. Examination reveals papilloedema but no focal signs. There are no abnormal findings on CT.

3   A 30-year-old man complains of a dull headache that is worse when lying down or when coughing. He has recently suffered a seizure.

4   A 65-year-old woman complains of a constant aching pain around the right eye radiating to the forehead. There is reduced vision in the eye, which is red and congested with a dilated pupil.

5   A 70-year-old woman complains of headache, drowsiness and unsteadiness over the last couple of days. On examination she is found to have papilloedema. She remembers falling over 3 weeks ago.

Answers: see page 91.

31 Weakness in the legs

A	myasthenia gravis	G	alcohol-induced neuropathy
B	Charcot–Marie–Tooth disease	H	Parkinson's disease
C	polymyalgia rheumatica	I	polymyositis
D	motor neuron disease	J	multiple sclerosis
E	Guillain–Barré syndrome	K	bilateral stroke
F	syringomyelia	L	neurofibromatosis

For each clinical scenario below, give the most likely cause for the clinical findings. Each option may be used only once.

1   A 60-year-old woman complains of bilateral proximal muscle weakness in the legs and dysphagia. On examination she has a purple rash on her cheeks.

2   A 40-year-old man presents with a recent history of progressive weakness in the arms and legs after an episode of diarrhoea. Examination revealed flaccid weakness of limbs with no reflexes.

3   A 55-year-old man presents with bilateral progressive worsening muscle weakness. There is marked wasting of lower limb muscles and very brisk lower limb reflexes. Sensation is normal.

4   A 13-year-old boy presents with bilateral pes cavus with clawing of the toes. There is atrophy of peroneal muscles and reduced reflexes and sensation distally.

5   A 30-year-old secretary presents with bilateral leg weakness and blurred vision. Fundoscopy reveals pale optic discs bilaterally.

Answers: see page 92.

32 Nerve lesions

A	radial nerve	H	L1
B	common peroneal nerve	I	C8, T1
C	S1	J	ulnar nerve
D	long thoracic nerve	K	median nerve
E	L2	L	posterior tibial nerve
F	T10	M	T12
G	S2		

Choose the most likely location of lesion that gives rise to the symptoms below. Each option may be used only once.

1   Inability to dorsiflex foot after blow to the side of knee.

2   Sensory loss over medial one and a half fingers.

3   A 25-year-old man presents with a winged scapula and the inability to raise his arm above the horizontal.

4   Sensory loss bilaterally below the level of the umbilicus.

5   Right-sided ptosis, miosis and wasting of small muscles of the right hand.

Answers: see page 94.

33 Cranial nerve lesions

A	V, VII, VIII, IX lesion	G	V lesion
B	right XII lesion	H	left XI lesion
C	left XII lesion	I	V, VII, VIII lesion
D	right XI lesion	J	IX, X lesion
E	IX lesion	K	VI lesion
F	IV, V, VII lesion	L	IV lesion

Which cranial nerve lesion(s) is(are) responsible for the symptoms and signs described below?

1   A 55-year-old man presents with unilateral weakness, wasting and fasciculation of the tongue. On examination the tongue deviates to the left on protrusion.

2   A 44-year-old man presents with progressive perceptive deafness, vertigo, unilateral facial weakness and loss of sensation on that side of the face. Imaging reveals the presence of a cerebellopontine tumour.

3   A patient complains of a hoarse voice, difficulty in swallowing and choking when drinking fluids. Examination reveals visible weakness of elevation of the palate, depression of palatal sensation and loss of the gag reflex.

4   A 28-year-old man presents after surgery with an inability to rotate the head to the right and to shrug the left shoulder.

5   A 35-year-old woman with multiple sclerosis complains of diplopia. Examination reveals inability to abduct pupil on one side.

Answers: see page 95.

34 Abnormal movements

A   tardive dyskinesia   G   hemiballismus
B   senile dystonia   H   Tourette's syndrome
C   myoclonus   I   tics
D   chorea   J   pill-rolling tremor
E   akathisia   K   torticollis
F   dysmetria   L   asterixis

Choose from the options above the term that describes the types of movement in the following clinical situations.

1   A jerky tremor of outstretched hands in an alcoholic with decompensated liver disease.

2   Non-rhythmic jerky purposeless movements in the hands of a 55-year-old man.

3   A 75-year-old man with poorly controlled diabetes is distressed by wild flinging of his right arm and right leg.

4   Grimacing and involuntary chewing in a 75-year-old woman on long-term treatment with neuroleptics.

5   Past-pointing in a 60-year-old woman being investigated for unsteady gait.

Answers: see page 95.

35 Neurological problems

A	muscular dystrophy	G	Sturge–Weber syndrome
B	Shy–Drager syndrome	H	syringomyelia
C	chronic fatigue syndrome	I	pseudobulbar palsy
D	neurofibromatosis	J	Bell's palsy
E	myasthenia gravis	K	cervical spondylisthesis
F	melanoma		

For each clinical scenario below, give the most likely cause for the clinical findings. Each option may be used only once.

1   A 45-year-old woman complains of a pain behind the right ear and that her mouth is sagging on the right-hand side.

2   A 62-year-old woman presents with a stiff spastic tongue and 'Donald Duck'-like speech. On examination she had a brisk jaw jerk and was prone to laughing inappropriately.

3   A 27-year-old woman presents with wasting and weakness of the small muscles of the hand. Examination reveals loss of pain and temperature sensation over the trunk and arms with intact vibration sense.

4   A 34-year-old woman complains of generalized weakness in her muscles, diplopia and weakening of her voice if talking for longer than 30 s. Examination reveals bilateral ptosis.

5   A 15-year-old boy is found to have several coffee-coloured patches on his body. Slit-lamp examination reveals the presence of Lisch nodules.

Answers: see page 96.

36 Gait

A   myopathic gait
B   cerebellar ataxia
C   femoral nerve injury
D   sciatic nerve injury
E   Alzheimer's dementia
F   Parkinson's disease

G   sensory ataxia
H   Pick's dementia
I   Huntington's disease
J   Sydenham's chorea
K   psychogenic gait
L   spastic gait

For each clinical scenario below, give the most likely cause for the gait that is observed. Each option can be used only once.

1   A 65-year-old man with a festinant, shuffling gait.

2   A 60-year-old woman walks with a drop foot and high-stepping gait shortly after hip replacement.

3   A 65-year-old man presents after a stroke with a stiff right leg that drags forward in an arc.

4   A broad-based high-stepping gait in a known alcoholic.

5   A broad-based unstable gait with veering to the right side.

Answers: see page 98.

37 Falls and loss of consciousness

A	micturition syncope	G	drop attack
B	postural hypotension	H	Menière's disease
C	vasovagal syncope	I	anxiety attack
D	carotid sinus syncope	J	hypoglycaemia
E	Stokes–Adams attack	K	epilepsy
F	vertebrobasilar ischaemia		

For each clinical scenario below, give the most likely cause for the clinical findings. Each option may be used only once.

1   A 70-year-old man complains of several blackouts and falls every day. The blackout lasts for several seconds and is preceded by palpitations.

2   A 65-year-old woman presented with attacks of sudden weakness of the legs causing her to fall to the ground. There is no loss of consciousness or confusion afterwards. She has not had any attacks for several months now.

3   A 21-year-old student presents with hyperventilation, tachycardia and lightheadedness and is brought to A&E after 'blacking out'.

4   A 34-year-old woman falls to the ground after hearing some bad news.

5   A 60-year-old woman who has recently started antihypertensive medication has a fall after getting out of bed.

Answers: see page 99.

38 Site of neurological lesion

A	left occipital lobe	G	substantia nigra
B	right cerebellar lobe	H	frontal lobe
C	medial longitudinal fasciculus (MLF)	I	left parietal lobe
		J	dominant temporal lobe
D	non-dominant temporal lobe	K	left cerebellar lobe
E	caudate nucleus	L	right parietal lobe
F	right occipital lobe	M	bilateral nerve VI lesion

Choose the most probable site of lesion in these clinical scenarios. Each option may be used only once.

1   A 75-year-old, right-handed woman is noted to ignore stimuli on the left side of her body.

2   A 65-year-old woman with suspected dementia is noted to be aggressive and sexually disinhibited.

3   A 65-year-old man has been unable to understand the ward staff over the last few days and speaks fluently in jargon that cannot be understood. His speech and language were previously normal.

4   A 34-year-old woman with multiple sclerosis is found to have bilateral internuclear ophthalmoplegia.

5   A 41-year-old man presents with dementia and irregular jerky movements of the trunk and limbs. His father suffered from a similar problem.

Answers: see page 100.

39 Antiepileptic drug therapy

A	carbamazepine	G	phenytoin
B	tiagabine	H	gabapentin
C	paraldehyde	I	primidone
D	diazepam	J	lamotrigine
E	sodium valproate	K	ethosuximide
F	phenobarbitone	L	vigabatrin

For each clinical scenario, select the most probable antiepileptic medication that is responsible for the adverse effects described. Each option may be used only once.

1   A 45-year-old woman on antiepileptic therapy complains of acne and increased facial hair growth. She is on no other medication.

2   A 25-year-old man presents with visual field defects 2 months after starting a new anticonvulsant therapy.

3   A 21-year-old woman presenting with status epilepticus complains of rectal irritation after being given an antiepileptic medication per rectum.

4   A 32-year-old woman on treatment for temporal lobe epilepsy complains of tremor, drowsiness and thinning hair. She is found to have mildly raised liver enzyme levels.

5   A 24-year-old man who has recently started adjunctive antiepileptic therapy complains of a rash with blisters in the mouth and flu symptoms.

Answers: see page 101.

40 Treatment of headache

A amitriptyline
B morphine
C timolol
D paracetamol
E prednisolone
F evacuation via burr hole
G propranolol

H high–dose aspirin and metoclopramide
I pethidine
J acetazolamide
K carbamazepine
L sumatriptan
M hydrocortisone

For each clinical scenario below, suggest the most appropriate treatment for the headache. Each option may be used only once.

1 A 52-year-old man with ischaemic heart disease requires treatment for an acute migraine attack that has not responded to paracetamol.

2 A 75 year old has a headache and painful red congested eye with a dilated non-responsive pupil.

3 A 65-year-old woman presents with a headache that has lasted a few weeks. She gets pain in her mouth during meals and her scalp is tender on palpation.

4 A 70-year-old woman requiring treatment for troubling trigeminal neuralgia.

5 A 29-year-old man with a skull fracture is suffering from very severe pain overlying the laceration to his head. He has been admitted for overnight observation.

Answers: see page 103.

41 Treatment of Parkinson's disease

A	clozapine	H	apomorphine
B	thalamotomy	I	nortriptyline
C	bromocriptine	J	domperidone
D	ondansetron	K	amantadine
E	carbidopa	L	entacapone
F	metoclopramide	M	haloperidol
G	benzhexol			

For each clinical scenario below, suggest the most appropriate management. Each option may be used only once.

1   Improvement of tremor in a 70-year-old patient with Parkinson's disease on treatment with levodopa.

2   Control of vomiting in a patient being treated for Parkinson's disease.

3   A 65-year-old man with Parkinson's disease cannot tolerate levodopa-based therapy despite careful titration.

4   A patient on therapy for Parkinson's disease requires urgent treatment for acute psychosis.

5   A 75-year-old man with severe Parkinson's disease with symptoms that remain uncontrolled on maximum oral therapy.

Answers: see page 104.

ANSWERS

28 Dizziness and vertigo

Answers: J F D B I

A 45-year-old woman presents with a left-sided facial palsy and vertigo. She has impaired hearing on her left side and a vesicular rash is
noted around her external auditory meatus.

J   Ramsay Hunt syndrome is the name attributed to herpes zoster infection
of the geniculate ganglion. The external auditory meatus receives some
sensory innervation from the facial (VII) nerve, hence the vesicular rash
over this area.
Aciclovir is the treatment of choice.

A 55-year-old man presents with a history of recurrent spontaneous
attacks of vertigo, hearing loss and tinnitus. These attacks last up to
2 h and are sometimes associated with vomiting.

F   Menière's disease is associated with the triad of vertigo, tinnitus and
deafness. The aetiology is unclear and some authorities suggest that it
may arise from a dilatation of the endolymphatic system. The vertigo
may be disabling and associated with vomiting. The deafness is of a sen-
sorineural nature. Rest is advised for acute attacks. Long-term prophylaxis involves the use of vestibular sedatives, e.g. cinnarizine or
betahistine, but results are disappointing.

A 65-year-old woman presents with vertigo, vomiting and dysphagia.
On examination there is a left-sided Horner's syndrome, and loss of
pain and temperature on the right side of the face.

D   The posterior inferior cerebellar artery (PICA) supplies the dorsal lateral
medullary plate and parts of the posterior medial cerebellum. PICA
thrombosis results in lesions affecting cranial nerves, descending tracts
and the cerebellum that are known collectively as 'lateral medullary
syndrome'.
Ipsilateral signs include:
- decreased pain and temperature sensation of the face (descending tract
  and nucleus of nerve V)
- palatal, vocal fold paralysis (nerve IX, X involvement)
- Horner's syndrome (sympathetic tract)
- cerebellar signs, e.g. ataxia, nystagmus.
Contralateral signs include:
- decreased pain and temperature sensation of the body (spinothalamic
  tract)
- lateral medullary syndrome, eponymously known as Wallenberg's
  syndrome.

A 50-year-old man presents with vertigo when rolling over quickly in bed, getting out of bed and bending over. His hearing is normal.

B Benign paroxysmal positional vertigo is characterized by short episodes of vertigo triggered by head movements. Patients often report problems when rolling over in bed/getting out of bed. It is caused by free-floating particles in the endolymph of the semicircular canal which in turn cause continuing stimulation of the auditory canal for several seconds after movement of the head has ceased.

Hallpike's manoeuvre is used to confirm the diagnosis of benign paroxysmal positional vertigo. The patient is asked to sit upright with the head facing the examiner. The examiner grasps the patient's head between his hands and rapidly moves the patient from a sitting to lying position with the head tipped below the horizontal plane, 45° to the side, and with the side of the affected ear (and semicircular canal) downwards.

A positive test provokes vertigo and rotatory nystagmus that typically has a latency of a few seconds before onset and fatigues after about 30 s. If the nystagmus appears immediately on performing the manoeuvre and does not fatigue, a cerebellar mass lesion may be responsible and computed tomography (CT) should be performed.

The condition can be treated with the Epley manoeuvre (orient the head in various positions to displace the particles from the posterior canal).

A 20-year-old man presents with vertigo having suffered with symptoms of flu for several days.

I Vestibular neuronitis is associated with a preceding infection/illness. The vertigo is severe and presents abruptly with vomiting but no deafness/tinnitus. The vertigo usually diminishes after a few days and in many cases there is complete recovery within a couple of weeks. Some individuals, however, develop benign paroxysmal positional vertigo afterwards.

29 Headache

Answers: F A L J B

A 40-year-old man complains of severe headache of sudden onset 4 h ago, likened to being kicked in the back of the head. He has vomited twice and is now feeling stiff in his neck.

F Subarachnoid haemorrhage is usually caused by rupture of berry aneurysms found on the circle of Willis. Disease states associated with high blood pressure, e.g. coarctation of aorta, polycystic disease or defective collagen synthesis, e.g. Ehlers–Danlos syndrome, predispose to berry aneurysm formation.

Typical symptoms are of a severe occipital headache that is sometimes likened to being 'kicked in the back of the head'.

Initial investigation of choice is a CT brain scan. However, findings can be negative in 10–15 per cent of subarachnoid haemorrhage. In patients in whom clinical suspicion is high and CT scan is negative, lumbar puncture (LP) should be performed.

Subarachnoid haemorrhage is confirmed by presence of xanthochromia resulting from denatured red blood cells within the cerebrospinal fluid (CSF). This can take up to 12 h to form and, therefore, LP should be delayed for at least 12 h after onset of headache. Discoloration of the CSF should be uniform, unlike a bloody tap where more red blood cells are present in the initial sample.

Some patients may present with a small sentinel bleed with minimal symptoms. It is important to make this diagnosis because timely intervention may prevent a more catastrophic later event.

A 40-year-old businesswoman complains of a headache that feels like a tight band around her head.

A   Tension headaches are common and the 'band-like' headache is a classic description. Diagnosis requires the absence of symptoms and signs of other types of headache. Treatment is rarely effective and avoidance of the precipitants, e.g. stress, is the best remedy. Chronic use of analgesics can lead to 'rebound headache' on withdrawal. Antidepressants are sometimes prescribed, although benefit is uncertain.

A 55-year-old woman presents with a headache that has lasted a few weeks. She gets pain in her jaw during meals and her scalp is tender on palpation.

L   Giant cell arteritis is a medium-sized vessel vasculitis. Classically it affects the temporal vessels giving symptoms of headache, scalp tenderness and jaw claudication. There is a risk of blindness if the disease is left untreated and treatment should be commenced empirically with oral corticosteroids.

Diagnosis can be confirmed with a temporal artery biopsy and the condition is usually associated with a high erythrocyte sedimentation rate (ESR)/C-reactive protein (CRP). CRP is always elevated, although ESR is very occasionally normal. As disease may not affect the part of the artery that has been biopsied, treatment should be continued even though the biopsy is negative if the clinical suspicion is high. Giant cell arteritis is recognized to overlap with polymyalgia rheumatica.

A 30-year-old man complains of rapid-onset pain around his left eye every night for the last 2 weeks, associated with lid swelling, watery eye and flushing. He suffers from these bouts every 3 months.

J   Cluster headache typically presents with recurrent brief attacks of headache around the eye. The hallmark of cluster headache is the association with autonomic symptoms and signs, e.g. nasal stuffiness, conjunctival hyperaemia, Horner's syndrome.

The clusters usually last between a few weeks and a few months.

A 24-year-old woman complains of a unilateral throbbing headache lasting 6 hours associated with vomiting and photophobia. She has had several episodes in the past.

B   The classic description of migraine includes a preceding aura before the onset of the headache, but this feature does not occur in most patients.

30 Headache

Answers: L G J D E

A 56-year-old woman complains of unilateral stabbing pain on the surface of her scalp and around her eye. The pain is precipitated by washing or touching the specific area.

L   This woman gives a classic history of trigeminal neuralgia affecting the ophthalmic division of the trigeminal nerve. This condition more commonly presents in the mandibular and maxillary branches. It is principally a complaint in older patients.

A 28-year-old woman complains of headache and double vision which is worse when lying down. Examination reveals papilloedema but no focal signs. There are no abnormal findings on CT.

G   Benign intracranial hypertension is a condition of unknown aetiology which usually affects obese women. Steroids and tetracyclines are recognized precipitants.
Diagnosis of raised CSF pressure is made by LP. Symptoms often resolve after LP. Chronic treatment includes the use of repeated LPs and diuretics.

A 30-year-old man complains of a dull headache that is worse when lying down or when coughing. He has recently suffered a seizure.

J   A description of early morning headache that is exacerbated by lying down/coughing/sneezing is a classic description of raised intracranial pressure. The development of seizures is a sinister finding and urgent imaging is warranted.

A 65-year-old woman complains of a constant aching pain around the right eye radiating to the forehead. There is reduced vision in the eye, which is red and congested with a dilated pupil.

D   Acute closed angle glaucoma mostly affects the long-sighted elderly population. It is caused by blockage of drainage of aqueous humour from the anterior chamber via the canal of Schlemm.
Stimuli that cause pupillary dilatation (e.g. sitting in the dark) increases the tightness of contact between the iris and the lens and can precipitate an attack.

A 70-year-old woman complains of headache, drowsiness and unsteadiness over the last couple of days. On examination she is found to have papilloedema. She remembers falling over 3 weeks ago.

E   There is not always a prior history of head injury. Alcohol abuse is a risk factor for chronic subdural haemorrhage. Neurosurgical opinion should be sought early, although many subdural haemorrhages can be handled conservatively because the bleeds clot spontaneously. The presence of papilloedema indicates that the subdural bleed is increasing the intracranial pressure. Initially the intracranial compliance is high and so the increase in volume caused by the developing bleed causes only small increases in intracranial pressure. However, this compliance decreases (compensatory mechanisms to cope with increases in pressure are limiting) and small increases in volume are associated with large increases in intracranial pressure. This is clinically important because patients may deteriorate very quickly and should therefore be regularly monitored.

31 Weakness in the legs

Answers: C E D B A

A 60-year-old woman complains of bilateral proximal muscle weakness in the legs and dysphagia. On examination she has a purple rash on her cheeks.

C   There are many non-neurological causes of weakness in the legs. Polymyositis is an autoimmune disease characterized by non-suppurative inflammation of skeletal muscle. In severe disease there can be respiratory muscle weakness and also cardiac involvement. Creatine kinase (CK) is usually markedly elevated. Electromyography (EMG) characteristically shows fibrillation potentials.

A 40-year-old man presents with a recent history of progressive weakness in the arms and legs after an episode of diarrhoea. Examination revealed flaccid weakness of limbs with no reflexes.

E   Guillain–Barré syndrome describes a presentation of an ascending polyneuropathy of unknown aetiology, which may be associated with a preceding infection. The weakness is symmetrical and may affect proximal muscles sooner than distal ones. Cranial nerves and the autonomic nervous system may also be involved. Involvement of respiratory muscles can be fatal and regular monitoring of vital capacity is important. In these cases it is often safer to initiate ventilation sooner rather than later. Sensory symptoms are usually mild with complaints of numbness and tingling in the limbs.
Intravenous immunoglobulin is often used to shorten the duration of the disease. Prognosis is good with over 85 per cent patients making a complete or near complete recovery.

A 55-year-old man presents with bilateral progressive worsening muscle weakness. There is marked wasting of lower limb muscles and very brisk lower limb reflexes. Sensation is normal.

D   Motor neuron disease (MND) is a progressive degenerative disease that affects the upper and lower motor neurons (LMNs). There is characteristically NO sensory involvement.

It is useful to be familiar with the following three common patterns of involvement:

(i)   Progressive muscular atrophy: anterior horn wasting lesion with wasting often beginning in the distal muscles of the hand and then spreading. Fasciculation is a common finding.

(ii)   Amyotrophic lateral sclerosis: involvement of the lateral corticospinal tract gives a progressive spastic teraparesis/paraparesis. The presence of LMN signs, e.g. wasting, fasciculation, differentiates this diagnosis from other causes of spastic weakness.

(iii)   Progressive bulbar palsy: the lower cranial nerve nuclei and their connections are primarily affected. Dysarthria and dysphagia are common symptoms. This pattern of disease is more common in women than in men.

A 13-year-old boy presents with bilateral pes cavus with clawing of the toes. There is atrophy of peroneal muscles and reduced reflexes and sensation distally.

B   Charcot–Marie–Tooth disease is a progressive peroneal muscle atrophy. There are both autosomal dominant and recessive inheritances observed in different families. Charcot–Marie–Tooth disease is now described as a hereditary sensorimotor neuropathy (HSMN) because several clinical variants have been identified associated with different gene defects. HSMN types I and II are the most common types.

HSMN type I is a demyelinating neuropathy of insidious onset presenting typically in the first decade of life with foot deformities (e.g. pes cavus), muscle weakness (distal weakness that affects legs earlier and more severely than arms) and loss of balance. The presence of foot drop results in frequent trips and falls.

HSMN type II usually presents later in the second decade of life. The weakness in distal lower limb muscles is often accompanied by distal sensory loss. Foot deformities are less marked than in type I disease and patients may even be completely asymptomatic.

A 30-year-old secretary presents with bilateral leg weakness and blurred vision. Fundoscopy reveals pale optic discs bilaterally.

 In this case the pale bilateral optic discs indicate previous subclinical episodes of optic neuritis. Multiple sclerosis (MS) is an inflammatory demyelinating disease of the central nervous system (CNS) that has a progressive course. There is an increased prevalence further away from the equator but the aetiology is still unknown. More women are affected (1.5–2:1).

Diagnosis is made clinically but magnetic resonance imaging (MRI) is the imaging of choice to detect demyelinating plaques. CSF examination usually shows oligoclonal bands of IgG on electrophoresis. Electrophysiological tests reveal delays in the propagation of potentials (e.g. visual, somatosensory, auditory evoked potentials).

Intravenous methylprednisolone can reduce the severity of relapses but does not improve long-term prognosis. Interferon-β has been shown to reduce the relapse rate in patients suffering from the relapsing–remitting form of the illness but its use is limited because of its high cost.

32 Nerve lesions

Answers: B J D F I

Inability to dorsiflex foot after blow to the side of knee.

B   The blow to the leg compresses the common peroneal nerve against the head of the fibula. There is a weakness in eversion and the presence of foot drop. There may be some numbness on the anterolateral aspect of the shin.

Sensory loss over medial one and a half fingers.

J   The median nerve supplies sensation to the palmar surface of the first three and a half fingers. In ulnar nerve palsy there may be features of a 'claw hand', i.e. hyperextension at the metacarpophalangeal joints and flexion at the interphalangeal joints of the fourth and fifth fingers.

A 25-year-old man presents with a winged scapula and the inability to raise his arm above the horizontal.

D   The long thoracic nerve supplies serratus anterior which allows the lateral and forward movement of the scapula.

Sensory loss bilaterally below the level of the umbilicus.

F   T10 is the level of the umbilicus

Right-sided ptosis, miosis and wasting of small muscles of the right hand.

I   This is often called a Klumpke's paralysis (C8–T1 lesion) with paralysis of the small muscles of the hand, arm held in adduction and lack of sensation over the ulnar side of the arm. The presence of a Horner's syndrome results from an avulsion of T1 (the preganglionic sympathetic fibres leave the spinal nerve soon after it emerges from the intervertebral foramen).

33 Cranial nerve lesions

Answers: C I J H K

A 55-year-old man presents with unilateral weakness, wasting and fasciculation of the tongue. On examination the tongue deviates to the left on protrusion.

C   Tongue deviates to the side of the lesion.

A 44-year-old man presents with progressive perceptive deafness, vertigo, unilateral facial weakness and loss of sensation on that side of the face. Imaging reveals the presence of a cerebellopontine tumour.

I   Cerebellopontine tumours often present clinically as a result of impingement on cranial nerves in the cerebellopontine angle.

A patient complains of a hoarse voice, difficulty in swallowing and choking when drinking fluids. Examination reveals visible weakness of elevation of the palate, depression of palatal sensation and loss of the gag reflex.

J   Cranial nerve IX and X lesions rarely occur in isolation and can also accompany nerve XI and XII lesions after infarction in the brain stem or as a result of pathology around the jugular foramen.

A 28-year-old man presents after surgery with an inability to rotate the head to the right and to shrug the left shoulder.

H   Accessory nerve is the motor supply to trapezius and sternocleido-mastoid. The latter muscle allows rotation of the head to the opposite side.

A 35-year-old woman with multiple sclerosis complains of diplopia. Examination reveals inability to abduct pupil on one side.

K   Diplopia in multiple sclerosis can result from demyelination of cranial nerves associated with eye movements, i.e. III, IV and VI.

34 Abnormal movements

Answers: L D G A F

A jerky tremor of outstretched hands in an alcoholic with decompensated liver disease.

L   This is elicited by asking the patient to 'stretch out your arms and cock your wrists back'.

Non-rhythmic jerky purposeless movements in the hands of a 55-year-old man.

D   Huntington's disease is an autosomal dominant condition resulting from a trinucleotide repeat mutation on the short arm of chromosome 4.

There is marked loss of neurons in the caudate nucleus and putamen. The patient usually presents in middle age with development of chorea. The condition is progressive and dementia may occur in the latter stages.

Tetrabenazine is often used to control the choreiform movements. Sydenham's chorea is a rare complication of rheumatic fever that involves onset of choreiform movements later in life.

A 75-year-old man with poorly controlled diabetes is distressed by wild flinging of his right arm and right leg.

G   Usually the underlying pathology is infarction/haemorrhage in the contralateral subthalamic nucleus.

Grimacing and involuntary chewing in a 75-year-old woman on long-term treatment with neuroleptics.

A   Tardive dyskinesia is a movement disorder that usually appears only after long-term treatment with typical antipsychotic medications and other drugs with dopamine antagonist activity, e.g. metoclopramide. Withdrawal of the responsible drug can lead to improvement but the condition is irreversible in some patients. Atypical antipsychotic medications such as clozapine and risperidone are less likely to cause extrapyramidal side effects and tardive dyskinesia.

Past-pointing in a 60-year-old woman being investigated for unsteady gait.

F   Dysdiadochokinesis (incoordination of rapidly alternating movement), nystagmus and intention tremor are signs of cerebellar disease that can be easily elicited/observed at the bedside.

35 Neurological problems

Answers: J I H E D

A 45-year-old woman complains of a pain behind the right ear and that her mouth is sagging on the right-hand side.

J   In a Bell's palsy (lower motor neuron lesion affecting cranial nerve VII) all the muscles on one half of the face are affected. There may also be loss of taste sensation on the anterior two-thirds of the tongue because the facial nerve supplies sensory innervation to that area via the chorda tympani.

Improvement and complete recovery are common. EMG can often be a good predictor of outcome. In an upper motor neuron lesion (caused by a cerebrovascular accident or CVA, for example) there is sparing of the forehead as a result of bilateral innervation. The patient will be able to raise both eyebrows.

A 62-year-old woman presents with a stiff spastic tongue and 'Donald Duck'-like speech. On examination she had a brisk jaw jerk and was prone to laughing inappropriately.

I   Pseudobulbar palsy is an upper motor neuron lesion caused by bilateral lesions of the lower cranial nuclei and can be associated with emotional lability. It is known to occur in multiple sclerosis, motor neuron disease and after bilateral strokes affecting the corticobulbar pathways.

A 27-year-old woman presents with wasting and weakness of the small muscles of the hand. Examination reveals loss of pain and temperature sensation over the trunk and arms with intact vibration sense.

H   Syringomyelia is the term used to describe the development of a fluid-filled cavity (syrinx) within the spinal cord. The condition may be associated with an Arnold–Chiari malformation.

The expansion of the syrinx compresses surrounding tracts, giving rise to a particular pattern of symptoms/signs that relates to the position of the tracts within the spinal cord.

The pain and temperature modalities are characteristically affected first as a result of compression of decussating spinothalamic fibres anteriorly in the ventral horns. This loss of pain and temperature sensation is often described as occurring in a 'cape' distribution (over trunk and arms). Wasting and weakness of hands and arms reflects involvement of cervical anterior horn cells.

Sensory loss can result in Charcot's joints (neuropathic joints damaged through loss of sensation). Involvement of the sympathetic trunk can give rise to Horner's syndrome.

The condition is gradually progressive and there is no known curative treatment. Patients with an Arnold–Chiari malformation may be treated with decompression at the foramen magnum to slow progression.

A 34-year-old woman complains of generalized weakness in her muscles, diplopia and weakening of her voice if talking for longer than half a minute. Examination reveals bilateral ptosis.

E   Myasthenia gravis (MG) is an acquired autoimmune disease characterized by muscle weakness and fatiguability resulting from the presence of anti-acetylcholine receptor antibodies.

MG is associated with other autoimmune disease, e.g. thyroid disease. The patient usually presents as a young adult with extraocular and bulbar muscle weakness. Weakness of the facial muscles is very common. Indeed bilateral facial weakness gives rise to the classic horizontal smile called a 'myasthenic snarl'. Neck weakness leads to the head drooping. Limb weakness is usually much more pronounced proximally.

Detection of anti-acetylcholine receptor antibodies is a reliable test for diagnosis of MG.

A test dose of an anticholinesterase, e.g. edrophonium, improves muscle power and can also be used to aid diagnosis.

Myasthenia gravis can be treated with the use of anticholinesterases (oral pyridostigmine is a popular drug) and oral corticosteroids (for immuno-suppression).

Be aware of Eaton–Lambert syndrome (a manifestation of bronchial small cell carcinoma) where there is defective release of acetylcholine at neuromuscular junctions giving rise to a myasthenic syndrome. In myasthenic syndrome the muscle strength increases and reflexes return with repeated contraction, unlike MG where repeated contraction gives rise to more weakness and a reduction of reflexes.

A 15-year-old boy is found to have several coffee-coloured patches on his body. Slit-lamp examination reveals the presence of Lisch nodules.

D   This is a presentation of type I neurofibromatosis (also known as von Recklinghausen's disease). It is an autosomal dominant condition characterized by decreased production of neurofibromin.

Diagnosis requires two of seven diagnostic criteria.

(i)   six or more café-au-lait spots >5 mm (in children <10) or >15 mm in adults

(ii)   axillary/inguinal freckling

(iii)   two or more neurofibromas or even one plexiform neurofibroma

(iv)   optic glioma

(v)   two or more Lisch nodules (iris hamartoma detected with slit-lamp examination)

(vi)   osseous lesion such as sphenoid dysplasia/pseudoarthrosis

(vii)   family history in first-degree relative.

36 Gait

Answers: F D L G B

A 65-year-old man with a festinant, shuffling gait.

F   There is a characteristic fixed stoop with reduced arm swing while walking. As a result of the impairment of righting reflexes, sufferers are sometimes observed to fall stiffly 'like a tree' without putting their arms out to break the fall.

A 60-year-old woman walks with a drop foot and high-stepping gait shortly after hip replacement.

D   Sciatic nerve is derived from the anterior primary rami of L4, L5, S1, S2 and S3, and divides into the common peroneal and tibial nerves about two-thirds of the way down the thigh.

Sciatic nerve injury is an important postoperative complication of hip replacement and can result from direct trauma or traction on the nerve.

There is lack of sensation over the lateral leg below the knee (and the entire sole of the foot) and inability to dorsiflex or evert the foot.

A 65-year-old man presents after a stroke with a stiff right leg that drags forward in an arc.

L   Strokes give rise to upper motor neuron lesions with weakness in a pyramidal distribution. The combination of spasticity in the leg extensors and weakness worse in the flexors of the lower limb gives rise to this spastic gait characterized by a stiff circumducted leg.

A broad-based high-stepping gait in a known alcoholic.

G   Sensory ataxia results from a loss of proprioception caused by peripheral neuropathy (in this case secondary to alcohol abuse). Romberg's test is used to identify proprioceptive sensory loss by demonstrating loss of postural control in darkness.
The patient is asked to stand with the feet together and to close his or her eyes. If the patient is unstable, the test is said to be positive. These patients sway and fall because they rely heavily on visual cues to maintain postural equilibrium. This test is not pathognomonic of proprioceptive loss because patients with bilateral vestibular damage and some patients with cerebellar disease require visual cues to keep their balance.

A broad-based unstable gait with veering to the right side.

B   Cerebellar disease affecting one hemisphere tends to cause the patient to veer towards the side of the lesion. If cerebellar disease affects the cerebellar midline vermis, there is truncal ataxia giving rise to difficulty in standing and even sitting on a stool unsupported.

37 Falls and loss of consciousness

Answers: E G I C B

A 70-year-old man complains of several blackouts and falls every day. The blackout lasts for several seconds and is preceded by palpitations.

E   A Stokes–Adam attack is caused by transient arrhythmias that decrease cardiac output sufficient to cause syncope. Both tachycardias and brady-cardias may be responsible. Recovery is typically quick. The patient is characteristically pale with the syncope and becomes flushed upon recovery.

A 65-year-old woman presented with attacks of sudden weakness of the legs causing her to fall to the ground. There is no loss of consciousness or confusion afterwards. She has not had any attacks for several months now.

G   There should be no loss of consciousness in drop attacks. The cause is unclear and they usually resolve spontaneously.

A 21-year-old student presents with hyperventilation, tachycardia and light-headedness and is brought to A&E after 'blacking out'.

I   Hyperventilation leads to a reduction in the Pa_{CO_2} and a respiratory alkalosis. Hypocapnic induced cerebral vessel vasoconstriction gives rise to the light-headedness and 'blacking out'.

Hyperventilation may be an appropriate response to a metabolic acidosis or as a response to primary CNS pathology affecting the brain stem. Hyperventilation can also occur as a means to increase Pa_{O_2} in a patient with asthma, chronic obstructive pulmonary disease (COPD), etc.

In this case hyperventilation has been provoked by anxiety and is characteristically associated with symptoms of lightheadedness, and circumoral and distal paraesthesia.

When a patient presents with a symptom of 'blacking out', it is important to find out exactly what he or she means by that term, i.e. loss of vision or loss of consciousness.

A 34-year-old woman falls to the ground after hearing some bad news.

C   Vasovagal syncope results from reflex bradycardia and peripheral vasodilatation in response to pain, emotion or prolonged standing. The patient may later report symptoms of nausea and closing in of the visual fields before collapse. The patient is unconscious for around 2 min and recovery is rapid in the supine position.

A 60-year-old woman who has recently started antihypertensive medication has a fall after getting out of bed.

B   Antihypertensive medication is a common cause of postural hypotension particularly in elderly people. This may occur as a result of hypovolaemia and/or autonomic dysfunction, e.g. diuretics may cause hypovolaemia and β blockers affect the autonomic nervous system. Other drug causes of autonomic dysfunction include L-dopa and tricyclic antidepressants.

38 Site of neurological lesion

Answers: L H J C E

A 75-year-old, right-handed woman is noted to ignore stimuli on the left side of her body.

L   This patient has sensory neglect suggesting a non-dominant hemisphere lesion. As the patient is right handed, we know that the dominant lobe must be on the left side, and hence the pathology is in the right parietal lobe.

The non-dominant lobe is largely responsible for visuospatial skills and this is reflected in the signs encountered, e.g. visual agnosia, dressing apraxia, constructional apraxia.

A 65-year-old woman with suspected dementia is noted to be aggressive and sexually disinhibited.

H   Socially and sexually disinhibited behaviour is a feature of frontal lobe lesions. Other signs include apathy, emotional lability, incontinence and perseveration.

A 65-year-old man has been unable to understand the ward staff over the last few days and speaks fluently in jargon that cannot be understood. His speech and language were previously normal.

J   This man is exhibiting signs of Wernicke's receptive dysphasia. His comprehension is impaired and his speech is fluent but full of jargon (that he is oblivious to). Look out for neologisms (in the absence of psychosis). A lesion in Broca's area (located in the dominant frontal lobe) gives rise to an expressive dysphasia, i.e. non-fluent speech with intact comprehension.

A 34-year-old woman with multiple sclerosis is found to have bilateral internuclear ophthalmoplegia.

C   Bilateral internuclear ophthalmoplegia is almost exclusively found in multiple sclerosis and is caused by bilateral involvement of the MLF. When the patient is asked to look towards the right, the left eye fails to adduct and the right eye develops coarse nystagmus in abduction. This is caused by the left MLF lesion.
When the patient is asked to look towards the left, the right eye fails to adduct and the left eye develops coarse nystagmus in abduction. This is caused by the right MLF lesion.

A 41-year-old man presents with dementia and irregular jerky movements of the trunk and limbs. His father suffered from a similar problem.

E   This is a presentation of Huntington's disease, an autosomal dominant condition, which usually presents in middle age. Pathologically, there is progressive degeneration of the striatum (caudate nucleus and putamen) and cerebral cortex (see Question 34, p. 95).

39 Antiepileptic drug therapy

Answers: G L C E J

A 45-year-old woman on antiepileptic therapy complains of acne and increased facial hair growth. She is on no other medication.

G   Phenytoin toxicity is associated with a 'cerebellar syndrome' (ataxia, nystagmus, intention tremor). Skin and collagen changes, including acne, hirsuitism and gum hypertrophy, have led to phenytoin becoming an unpopular drug, especially among younger patients. Phenytoin may also cause a folate-deficiency macrocytic anaemia.

A 25-year-old man presents with visual field defects 2 months after starting a new anticonvulsant therapy.

L   Vigabatrin is reserved for the treatment of epilepsy that is not satisfactorily controlled by other drugs. It has also been used as monotherapy in the treatment of West's syndrome (infantile spasms). Visual field defects are common and careful monitoring for this adverse effect is required. Unfortunately, in many cases these defects can persist even after treatment is discontinued.

A 21-year-old woman presenting with status epilepticus complains of rectal irritation after being given an antiepileptic medication per rectum.

C   Intravenous benzodiazepines are the usual first-line drug treatment of choice in status epilepticus. Paraldehyde is a useful drug for the treatment of status epilepticus because it causes little respiratory depression. It is associated with rectal irritation when delivered rectally as an enema. Diazepam injected intravenously is associated with a high risk of venous thrombophlebitis and so emulsion preparations are available to limit this. Intravenous lorazepam is also a popular choice in the treatment of major status epilepticus. It has the advantage of a longer duration of action than diazepam but it also has a slower onset of action.

A 32-year-old woman on treatment for temporal lobe epilepsy complains of tremor, drowsiness and thinning hair. She is found to have mildly raised liver enzyme levels.

E   Sodium valproate inhibits the activity of cytochrome P450 enzymes and thus will potentiate the activity of any drugs that are metabolized by these enzymes. Liver function must be monitored before and during the first few months of therapy. Valproate is contraindicated in active liver disease.

A 24-year-old man who has recently started adjunctive antiepileptic therapy complains of a rash with blisters in the mouth and flu symptoms.

J   Patients being treated with lamotrigine are warned to seek medical advice if a rash/flu-like symptoms develop. The risk of developing skin problems such as Stevens–Johnson syndrome and toxic epidermal necrolysis may be increased if lamotrigine is used with sodium valproate.

40 Treatment of headache

Answers: H J E K D

> A 52-year-old man with ischaemic heart disease requires treatment for an acute migraine attack that has not responded to paracetamol.

H   Aspirin and metoclopramide provide relief for the symptoms of pain and nausea/vomiting associated with migraine. The use of serotonin $5HT_1$ agonists such as sumatriptan are indicated if the patient fails to respond to conventional analgesics. Remember that the $5HT_1$ agonists are contraindicated in patients with coronary artery disease, previous myocardial infarction (MI) and uncontrolled hypertension.

> A 75 year old has a headache and painful red congested eye with a dilated non-responsive pupil.

J   This is a presentation of acute glaucoma and is a medical emergency because there is a risk of blindness. The symptoms are often precipitated/made worse by the dark. The severe pain can lead to nausea and vomiting. Acetazolamide acts by decreasing the formation of aqueous humour. After the intraocular pressure has been reduced, surgical intervention in the form of peripheral iridectomy can prevent recurrence.

> A 65-year-old woman presents with a headache that has lasted a few weeks. She gets pain in her mouth during meals and her scalp is tender on palpation.

E   Her symptoms and signs are suggestive of temporal/giant cell arteritis (GCA). The erythrocyte sedimentation rate (ESR) is characteristically very high in this condition. Treatment of choice is high-dose oral prednisolone. Skip lesions occur in temporal arteritis and so a negative temporal artery biopsy is not an indication to stop treatment in the face of high clinical suspicion of GCA.

> A 70-year-old woman requiring treatment for troubling trigeminal neuralgia.

K   Carbamazepine is commonly used to treat trigeminal neuralgia. Phenytoin and gabapentin have also been used to treat this condition. Cases refractory to medical treatment may be considered for surgery.

> A 29-year-old man with a skull fracture is suffering from very severe pain overlying the laceration to his head. He has been admitted for overnight observation.

D   Morphine causes pupillary constriction and should not be given as analgesia in this case of head injury because it will interfere with neurological observations.

41 Treatment of Parkinson's disease

Answers: G J C A H

> Improvement of tremor in a 70-year-old patient with Parkinson's disease on treatment with levodopa.

G   Benzhexol is a muscarinic acetylcholine receptor antagonist that is useful in treatment of parkinsonian tremor. Such anti-muscarinics are useful in treating tremor and rigidity, and in reducing sialorrhoea, but they have little effect on bradykinesia.

> Control of vomiting in a patient being treated for Parkinson's disease.

J   Domperidone is the antiemetic of choice because it does not penetrate the blood–brain barrier and can be given with centrally acting dopamine agonists to counteract their emetogenic effect.

> A 65-year-old man with Parkinson's disease cannot tolerate levodopa-based therapy despite careful titration.

C   Bromocriptine is a dopamine receptor agonist and is indicated if levodopa therapy is felt to be no longer adequate or if the patient cannot tolerate levodopa therapy. The use of bromocriptine is limited by its adverse effects, which include hypotension and fibrotic reactions, e.g. pulmonary fibrosis.

> A patient on therapy for Parkinson's disease requires urgent treatment for acute psychosis.

A   The dose of the responsible anti-parkinsonian drug should be reduced. Clozapine is an atypical antipsychotic and is thus preferred to the typical antipsychotics which have more marked extrapyramidal side effects.

> A 75-year-old man with severe Parkinson's disease with symptoms that remain uncontrolled on maximum oral therapy.

H   Apomorphine by subcutaneous injection/infusion is indicated if motor symptoms of Parkinson's disease remain refractory to maximal therapy with levodopa and other anti-parkinsonian drugs. Hospital admission is required for initiation of treatment. Adverse effects of nausea and vomiting are very common and so pre-treatment with domperidone is standard.

REVISION BOXES

Neurology

Box 1 summarizes some features of different causes of headache.

Box 1 Headache: classic presentation in an EMQ [29, 30]

Symptoms	Headache type
• Stress, tight band around head	Tension headache
• Sudden onset, 'kicked in back of head'; associated with vomiting	Subarachnoid haemorrhage
• Unilateral 'throbbing', aura, vomiting, photophobia	Migraine
• Tender pulseless temporal arteries; jaw claudication	Giant-cell arteritis
• Pain worse on coughing/sneezing; confusion, seizures, localizing focal neurology; signs of intracranial pressure, e.g. papilloedema	Mass lesion
• Usually obese young woman; ↑ CSF (cerebrospinal fluid) pressure but no mass lesion	Benign intracranial hypertension
• Fever, neck stiffness, photophobia, rash	Meningitis
• Head injury, chronic course fluctuating consciousness	Subdural haemorrhage

Discriminating an upper motor neuron lesion (UMN) from a lower motor neuron (LMN) lesion helps to exclude options in an EMQ (Box 2).

Box 2 Distinguishing UMN and LMN lesions

UMN lesion	LMN lesion
• Involves corticospinal tract • Weakness in upper limb extensors, lower limb flexors (pyramidal distribution) • Increased tone • Hyperreflexia, clonus • Pronator drift • Loss of abdominal reflexes • Extensor plantar response	• Lesion at level of anterior horn cell or distal to it • Fasciculation and wasting • Loss reflexes • Hypotonia

Box 3 summarizes some features of neurological disease that you may find in the scenarios of EMQs.

Box 3 Neurological disease

Signs	Disease
• Mixed UMN and LMN signs NO sensory loss	Motor neuron disease [31]

• Optic neuritis is a common finding
  in EMQs
  Non-specific signs, e.g. leg weakness,
  ataxia
  May mention heat worsens symptoms
  ↑↑ CSF protein, oligoclonal IgG bands
  on electrophoresis
  Delayed visual/somatosensory evoked
  potentials
	Multiple sclerosis [31]

• Lead-pipe rigidity, cog-wheel rigidity
  (if tremor)
  Pill rolling tremor
  Festinant gait with poor arm swing
	Parkinson's disease [36, 41]

• Young woman presents with weakness
  muscles
  On examination: bilateral ptosis,
  proximal muscle weakness
  Electromyography (EMG): decreased
  muscle action potential after continuous
  stimulation
  Serum acetylcholine receptor antibodies
	Myasthenia gravis [35]

• Onset of chorea in middle age,
  dementia later
  Positive family history (autosomal
  dominant)
	Huntington's disease [34, 38]

• Triad of: gait apraxia
     plus confusion
     plus incontinence
	Normal pressure hydrocephalus

Box 4 describes features of various neurological eponymous syndromes that may help you when answering EMQs.

Box 4 Features of eponymous syndromes

Feature	Syndrome
• Saddle anaesthesia Bowel/bladder disturbance Bilateral pain legs	Cauda equina syndrome
• Ipsilateral pyramidal signs plus contralateral loss of pain and temperature	Brown–Séquard syndrome
• Ascending symmetrical flaccid muscle weakness Preceding recent respiratory/ gastrointestinal infection	Guillain–Barré syndrome [31, 96]
• Combination of parkinsonism plus primary autonomic failure, e.g. postural hypotension	Shy–Drager syndrome
• Triad of: nystagmus, ophthalmoplegia, ataxia Caused by thiamine (vitamin B$_1$) deficiency Reversible but if untreated develops to Korsakoff's syndrome	Wernicke's encephalopathy [79, 99]
• Signs of gross defect in memory of recent events Confabulation may be present Condition is irreversible	Korsakoff's syndrome

Description of the patient's gait is often a good clue to a particular option in an EMQ (Box 5).

Box 5 Gait and different conditions [36]

Gait	Condition
Shuffling, festinant gait	Parkinson's disease
High-stepping/stamping gait	Sensory ataxia, e.g. peripheral neuropathy
Scissor gait	Spastic paraplegia
Wide-based gait	Cerebellar lesion
Shuffling small steps	Cerebrovascular disease (marche à la petit pas)

You will frequently come across an EMQ that tests knowledge of nerve root innervation and understanding of the level of a lesion when particular symptoms/signs are described (Box 6).

Box 6 Symptoms/signs of nerve root innervation

Reflexes	Movements
C5–C6 supinator	C5 – shoulder abduction
C5–C6 biceps	C5, C6 – elbow flexion
C7 triceps	C7 – elbow extension
L3–L4 knee	T1 – finger abduction
S1 ankle	L1, L2 – hip flexion
	L3, L4 – knee extension
	L4, L5 – dorsiflex ankle
	L5–S1 – hip extension
	S1 – knee flexion, plantar flexion and eversion ankle

An EMQ may describe a scenario and give a particular description of the patient's pupil(s) (Box 7). It is useful to be familiar with the main causes of such changes.

Box 7 The pupil in neurological problems

Description of pupil	Problem
Bilateral dilated pupils:	
• *plus* no vestibulo-ocular reflexes	Brain-stem death
• *plus* euphoric	Amphetamines, cocaine
• *plus* anticholinergic signs, e.g. ↑ pulse, ↓ BP, urinary retention	Tricyclic antidepressant overdose
Bilateral, pinpoint pupils:	
• with respiratory depression	Opiate overdose
Dilated pupil:	
• ptosis, eye deviated laterally and downwards	Nerve III lesion
• irregular, reacts poorly to light and accommodation	Myotonic pupil
• usually young woman may have reduced tendon reflexes	(Holmes–Adie pupil)
Constricted pupil:	
• irregular pupils, reacts to accommodation but not light (known as Argyll Robertson pupil)	Neurosyphilis
• unilateral ptosis, loss of sweating on same side of face (anhidrosis)	Horner's syndrome

Box 8 summarizes areas that are frequently tested in EMQs:
• The features of cranial nerve palsies that affect extraocular muscle movement.
• The likely site of lesion when a particular visual defect is described.

Box 8 Limited movements and visual field defects

Limited movements (caused by cranial nerve injury)	Lesion
• Defective elevation, depression, adduction	Nerve III lesion
• Defective depression in adduction Vertical diplopia worse in downgaze	Nerve IV lesion
• Failure to abduct Horizontal diplopia worse on abduction	Nerve VI lesion

Visual field defects	Lesion
• Bitemporal hemianopia	Chiasma lesion, e.g. pituitary tumour
• Superior quadrantanopia	Temporal lobe lesion
• Inferior quadrantanopia	Parietal lobe lesion
• Homonymous hemianopia	Optic radiation, visual cortex injury
• Central scotoma	Macula (e.g. degeneration/oedema)

Questions that test knowledge of clinical anatomy with respect to nerve injury are common in neurology EMQs (Box 9).

Box 9 Nerve injury [32]

Feature	Nerve
• Wasting thenar eminence Loss of sensation on lateral palmar surface of three and a half digits Test for weakness in abductor pollicis brevis Frequently affected in carpal tunnel syndrome	Median nerve (C6–T1)
• Wasting hypothenar eminence Sensory loss over medial one and a half fingers Test for weakness of abductor digiti minimi 'Claw hand' deformity	Ulnar nerve (C8–T1)
• Weakness of wrist extension, leading to 'wrist drop' Anaesthesia over first dorsal interosseous muscle	Radial nerve (C5–T1)
• Weakness in dorsiflexion and eversion of foot Sensory loss over dorsum of foot	Common peroneal nerve (L4–S1)
• Inability to invert foot or stand on tip-toe Sensory loss over sole of foot	Tibial nerve (L4–S3)

continued overleaf

continued
- Paralysis of intrinsic muscles of the hand   Klumpke's palsy [32]
  Loss of sensation in ulnar
  distribution (C8, T1)
  Horner's syndrome sometimes present
- Loss of shoulder abduction and elbow flexion   Erb's palsy (C5, C6)
  Arm held internally rotated
  'Waiter's tip' sign if arm adducted behind back

An EMQ may require you to establish the area of the brain that has been affected/vessels involved in a stroke (Box 10).

Box 10 Stroke: symptoms and signs

Symptoms/signs	Site of stroke
• Unilateral weakness/sensory deficit Homonymous hemianopia Higher cerebral dysfunction, e.g. dysphasia, neglect	Anterior circulation stroke
• Cranial nerve palsies/cerebellar signs, e.g. vertigo, dysarthria, ataxia, choking Isolated homonymous hemianopia	Posterior circulation stroke
• Patient can understand you but replies in non-fluent speech	Site: dominant frontal lobe (Broca's area) Broca's (expressive) dysphasia
• Patient has impaired comprehension Speech is fluent with jargon	Site: dominant temporoparietal lobe Wernicke's (receptive) dysphasia [38]
• Patient has symptoms of: – vertigo – vomiting – dysphagia	Site: PICA thrombosis Lateral medullary syndrome [28]
• Ipsilateral signs can include: – ataxia – Horner's syndrome – nerve V, VI palsy	
• Contralateral signs can include loss of pain, temperature and sensation in face	

SECTION 5: ORTHOPAEDICS AND RHEUMATOLOGY

QUESTIONS

42 Arthritis

A psoriatic arthritis
B discoid lupus erythematosus
C rheumatoid arthritis
D polymyalgia rheumatica
E systemic lupus erythematosus
F cervical spondylosis
G lumbar spondylosis

H Reiter's syndrome
I Sjögren's syndrome
J ankylosing spondylosis
K septic arthritis
L gout
M osteoporosis
N osteoarthritis

For each clinical scenario below, give the most likely cause for the clinical findings. Each option may be used only once.

1   A 54-year-old woman presents to her GP with swollen painful hands and feet, which are stiffer in the mornings. On examination there are signs of ulnar deviation and subluxation at the metacarpophalangeal (MCP) joints.

2   A 65-year-old woman complains of pain in her fingers on movement, which is worst at the end of the day. On examination there is joint tenderness and bony lumps at the distal interphalangeal (DIP) joints. A radiograph shows loss of joint space.

3   A 30-year-old woman complains of joint pain in her hands and feet. Her chest radiograph shows reduced lung volumes.

4   A 22-year-old man presents with an acute arthritis of the left knee, dysuria and bilateral conjunctivitis. He has recently suffered from gastroenteritis.

5   A 45-year-old woman presents with bilateral painful deformed DIP joints. Examination reveals discoloration and onycholysis of the nails.

Answers: see page 124.

43 Joint pain

A   psoriatic arthritis
B   polymyositis
C   rheumatoid arthritis
D   polymyalgia rheumatica
E   systemic lupus erythematosus
F   haemarthrosis
G   lumbar spondylosis

H   Reiter's syndrome
I   osteosarcoma
J   pseudogout
K   septic arthritis
L   gout
M   osteoporosis
N   osteoarthritis

For each clinical scenario below, give the most likely cause for the clinical findings. Each option may be used only once.

1   A 64-year-old patient who has recently been started on medication for hypertension presents with a very painful, hot, swollen metatarsophalangeal joint.

2   A 12-year-old haemophiliac presents to A&E with severe pain after falling over and banging his right knee.

3   A 55-year-old man presents to A&E with fever and an exquisitely painful right knee. On examination his right knee is red, hot and swollen. Purulent fluid is aspirated from the joint.

4   A 60-year-old woman presents with a painful swollen knee. Her radiograph shows chondrocalcinosis and joint aspiration reveals presence of weakly positive birefringent crystals.

5   A 65-year-old woman presents with a 1-month history of pain and stiffness in her shoulders, worse in the mornings. She says that she was treated in hospital last year for headache and jaw pain.

Answers: see page 125.

44 Pain in the hip

A   slipped femoral epiphysis   H   septic arthritis
B   osteoarthritis   I   fractured sacroiliac joint
C   congenital dislocation of hip   J   fractured neck femur
D   fracture pubic ramus   K   Charcot joint
E   transient synovitis   L   idiopathic growth retardation
F   tuberculous arthritis   M   Perthes' disease
G   rheumatoid arthritis

For each clinical scenario below, give the most likely cause for the clinical find-ings. Each option may be used only once.

1   An obese 12-year-old boy presents with pain in his right hip. On examination the hip is flexed, abducted and externally rotated. His mother has suffered from TB in the past.

2   A 6-year-old boy presents with a pain in the hip and a limp. All movements at the hip are limited. His radiograph shows decrease in size of the nuclear femoral head with patchy density.

3   A 3-year-old girl presents to the orthopaedic clinic with a waddling gait. Her mother says that there has been a delay in walking. On examination there is an extra crease on the left thigh.

4   An 80-year-old woman presents to A&E after a fall. On examination the left hip is adducted, externally rotated and excruciatingly painful.

5   An 8-year-old boy presents to A&E with marked limping and pain in the right hip, which resolves within 48 h. His radiographs show no abnormality at the hip or other joint involvement. Bone scan 2 weeks later is also normal. The patient's mother suffers from osteoarthritis.

Answers: see page 126.

45 Back pain

A   Paget's disease
B   polymyositis
C   Scheuermann's disease
D   vertebral disc prolapse
E   osteomyelitis
F   Reiter's disease

G   myeloma
H   rheumatoid arthritis
I   Pott's disease
J   spinal stenosis
K   ankylosing spondylitis

For each clinical scenario below, give the most likely cause for the clinical findings. Each option may be used only once.

1   A 22-year-old man complains of stiffness in the lower back and buttock pain that is relieved by exercise. He also suffers from bouts of painful red eye. His ESR is raised. His radiograph shows blurring of the upper vertebral rims of the lumbar spine.

2   A 60-year-old woman presents with constant backache. Her ESR and serum calcium are markedly elevated.

3   A 65-year-old man with osteoarthritis complains of back pain worse on walking along, with aching and heaviness in both legs that force him to stop walking. Pain is relieved slowly after rest or leaning forward.

4   A 13-year-old girl complains of backache and fatigue. She is worried that she is becoming increasingly round-shouldered. On examination, she has a smooth thoracic kyphosis. Her radiograph shows wedge-shaped vertebral bodies in the thoracic spine.

5   A 35-year-old tourist complains of severe back pain with inability to straighten up after lifting a suitcase yesterday. He now presents with weakness of his big toe extension and loss of sensation on the outer side of the calf.

Answers: see page 127.

46 Rheumatological conditions

A	polymyositis	G	ankylosing spondylitis
B	Behçet's disease	H	systemic sclerosis
C	syphilis	I	Stevens–Johnson's syndrome
D	relapsing polychondritis	J	rheumatoid arthritis
E	polymyalgia rheumatica	K	Sjögren's syndrome
F	primary Raynaud's disease	L	Reiter's syndrome

For each clinical scenario below, give the most likely cause for the clinical findings. Each option may be used only once.

1   A 45-year-old woman complains of cold numb fingers and difficulty in swallowing. On examination she has tight skin, thickening of the fingers and telangiectasia.

2   A 51-year-old woman complains of weakness in her shoulders and thighs. She has a significantly raised creatine kinase (CK) level.

3   A 25-year-old man has been referred to rheumatology clinic with multiple painful stiff joints and uveitis. He also complains of ulcers on his penis and mouth.

4   A 45-year-old woman presents with dryness in the eyes and mouth. Her Schirmer's test is positive.

5   A patient presents to rheumatology clinic with recurrent attacks of pain and swelling in the nose and external ear.

Answers: see page 128.

47 Complications of fractures

A	compartment syndrome	G	delayed union
B	osteoporosis	H	Sudeck's atrophy
C	pneumothorax	I	malunion
D	ulnar nerve injury	J	myositis ossificans
E	pulmonary embolus	K	haemarthrosis
F	median nerve injury	L	radial nerve injury

For each clinical scenario below, give the most likely cause for the clinical findings. Each option may be used only once.

1   A 25-year-old man presents with a blue right arm with absent radial pulse and painful passive finger extension after a supracondylar fracture of humerus.

2   A 40-year old woman presents 5 weeks after a radial fracture with a painful swollen hand. The hand is cold and cyanosed with heightened temperature sensitivity.

3   A 70-year-old woman complains of right-sided pleuritic chest pain 10 days after a fractured neck of femur.

4   A 60-year-old woman complains of pain, swelling and reduced mobility 4 months after suffering a fractured neck of femur. Her radiograph shows absence of callus at fracture site.

5   A 65-year-old woman who falls on an outstretched arm shows weakness of wrist extensors.

Answers: see page 130.

48 Management of fractures

A   skin traction
B   collar-and-cuff sling
C   broad sling
D   plaster from wrist to above knuckle
E   gallows' traction
F   internal fixation
G   rest and mobilization
H   manipulation under local anaesthesia and cast
I   bone traction
J   plaster from below elbow to above knuckle
K   analgesia + weight-bearing

For each clinical scenario below, suggest the most appropriate management. Each option may be used only once.

1   A 24-year-old man presents with a swollen painful hand after a falling over playing squash. His radiograph reveals a scaphoid fracture.

2   A 1-year-old baby requires traction after fracture of the right femur.

3   A 65-year-old woman requires treatment for displaced fractured neck of femur.

4   A 35-year-old woman presents after a fall on an outstretched arm. Her radiograph shows an undisplaced transverse fracture of the right humerus.

5   A 75-year-old woman suffers a displaced Colles' fracture.

Answers: see page 131.

49 Fall on the outstretched hand

A	Colles' fracture	G	Galeazzi's fracture
B	scapular fracture	H	fracture clavicle
C	posterior dislocation shoulder	I	Monteggia's fracture
D	olecranon fracture	J	supracondylar fracture
E	anterior dislocation shoulder	K	fractured humeral shaft
F	scaphoid fracture	L	Smith's fracture

For each clinical scenario below, suggest the most likely injury that has resulted. Each option may be used only once.

1   A 24-year-old woman presents with pain on wrist movements after a fall on to her hand. On examination there is tenderness and swelling in the anatomical snuffbox.

2   A 68-year-old woman presents with fracture at distal radial head with dorsal displacement of distal fragment after a fall.

3   A 7-year-old boy presents with a swollen painful elbow after a fall. He is unable to move the arm because of the pain.

4   A 19-year-old rugby player falls on a backward stretched hand and presents with loss of shoulder contour and absent sensation on a patch below the shoulder.

5   A 40-year-old woman presents after a fall on an outstretched hand with wrist drop.

Answers: see page 131.

50 Shoulder problems

A	ruptured long head of biceps	G	posterior dislocation shoulder
B	Sprengel's shoulder	H	anterior dislocation shoulder
C	tendonitis, long head of biceps	I	fracture clavicle
D	osteoarthritis	J	fractured neck of humerus
E	impingement syndrome	K	adhesive capsulitis
F	rheumatoid arthritis	L	fractured scapula

For each clinical scenario below, give the most likely cause for the clinical findings. Each option may be used only once.

1   A 21-year-old woman presents with a very painful shoulder locked in medial rotation after an epileptic fit.

2   A 55-year-old man complains of shoulder pain aggravated in abduction of arm between 60° and 120°.

3   A 30-year-old bodybuilder presents with an aching shoulder. Flexing elbow reveals a prominent lump in the upper arm.

4   A 50-year-old man complains of a 9-month history of stiffness in the shoulder. The shoulder was originally extremely painful but now only the stiffness remains.

5   A 65-year-old woman presents with shoulder pain and restricted movement in all directions. Her radiograph shows reduced joint space and subchondral sclerosis.

Answers: see page 133.

51 Knee problems

A	genu varum	G	dislocation of patella
B	collateral ligament rupture	H	genu valgum
C	suprapatellar bursitis	I	osteoarthritis
D	Baker's cyst	J	anterior cruciate ligament tear
E	pre–patellar bursitis	K	meniscal cyst
F	meniscal tear	L	Osgood–Schlatter disease

For each clinical scenario below, give the most likely cause for the clinical findings. Each option may be used only once.

1   A 22-year-old figure-skater presents with a painful locked knee with limited extension after a twisting injury.

2   A 24-year-old footballer presents with a painful knee after a tackle from behind. With the quadriceps relaxed, the anterior glide of the tibia on the femur is 1.0 cm.

3   A 14-year-old girl successfully treated for rickets 3 years ago shows bow-legged deformity.

4   A 16-year-old boy complains of a painful knee after exercise and a tender lump over the tibial tuberosity.

5   A 50-year-old carpet layer presents with a swelling directly over the patella. The joint is normal.

Answers: see page 134.

52 Management of painful joints

A exercise and physiotherapy
B paracetamol
C allopurinol
D colchicine
E high-dose aspirin
F oral penicillin
G oral prednisolone

H intravenous flucloxacillin, oral fusidic acid
I intravenous hydrocortisone
J sulfasalazine (sulphasalazine)
K ibuprofen
L methotrexate

For each clinical scenario below, suggest the most appropriate management. Each option may be used only once.

1 A 24-year-old man presented with lower back pain and stiffness that was worse in the morning. He has a question-mark posture.

2 An 80-year-old man with a 30-year history of rheumatoid arthritis presents to A&E with fever and pain in the right knee. On examination his right knee is red, hot and swollen. Aspirated synovial fluid is frankly purulent.

3 A 65-year-old woman recently diagnosed with osteoarthritis requires medication for joint pain.

4 A 64-year-old woman who has been successfully treated for acute gout requires prophylactic medication.

5 A 65-year-old woman with polymyalgia rheumatica.

Answers: see page 134.

53 Disease-modifying anti-rheumatic drugs (DMARDs)

A   penicillamine
B   sulfasalazine (sulphasalazine)
C   ciclosporin
D   mebeverine
E   hydroxychloroquine
F   anti-TNF (tumour necrosis
     factor) therapy

G   ibuprofen
H   methotrexate
I   prednisolone
J   diclofenac
K   gold

Select the medication, from the above options, that is most likely to be responsible for the adverse effects in the patients on DMARDs presenting in the questions below.

1   Computed tomography (CT) of patient on long-term DMARD treatment shows pulmonary and hepatic fibrosis.

2   Fertility testing reveals oligospermia in a 48-year-old man on DMARD treatment.

3   A patient complains of grossly swollen gums.

4   A patient taking an intramuscular DMARD presents with an itchy erythematous rash covering the whole body.

5   A 65-year-old woman patient presents with gross irreversible retinopathy.

Answers: see page 135.

ANSWERS

42 Arthritis

Answers: C N E H A

A 54-year-old woman presents to her GP with swollen painful hands and feet, which are stiffer in the mornings. On examination there are signs of ulnar deviation and subluxation at the MCP joints.

C   Ulnar deviation and subluxation of MCP joints are signs of advanced disease. Swelling of the fingers (sausage-like) and MCP joint swelling are earlier signs.

A 65-year-old woman complains of pain in her fingers on movement, which is worst at the end of the day. On examination there is joint tenderness and bony lumps at the DIP joints. A radiograph shows loss of joint space.

N   The radiological changes of osteoarthritis include loss of joint space, subchondral sclerosis, osteophytes and subchondral cyst formation. Osteophytes at the proximal interphalangeal and DIP joints are called Bouchard's and Heberden's nodes respectively. Previous joint damage is a risk factor for the development of osteoarthritic disease. Simple analgesics such as paracetamol should be prescribed for pain relief rather than long courses of non-steroidal anti-inflammatory drugs (NSAIDs) (risk of gastrointestinal bleeding with prolonged use).

A 30-year-old woman complains of joint pain in her hands and feet. Her chest radiograph shows reduced lung volumes.

E   Systemic lupus erythematosus (SLE) is an inflammatory multisystemic disorder that is nine times more common in women than in men. The joints are most often affected in a symmetrical fashion with no bony erosion (unlike rheumatoid arthritis). Rarely, there may be markedly deformed joints caused by joint laxity that resemble rheumatoid arthritis (Jaccoud's arthropathy).
Lung involvement occurs in up to half of patients with SLE. Manifestations include pleuritic chest pain, pleural effusions (these are common and often bilateral), acute/chronic pneumonitis and the rare 'shrinking lung syndrome'.

A 22-year-old man presents with an acute arthritis of the left knee, dysuria and bilateral conjunctivitis. He has recently suffered from gastroenteritis.

H   Reiter's disease involves a triad of urethritis, conjunctivitis and seronegative arthritis. Joint symptoms may be the presenting complaint. It is often

triggered by an infection, e.g. a sexually transmitted infection or gastroenteritis. Cutaneous manifestations include keratoderma blenorrhagica,
circinate balanitis and mouth ulcers. Enthesitis causing plantar fasciitis is
also well recognized.

**A 45-year-old woman presents with bilateral painful deformed DIP
joints. Examination reveals discoloration and onycholysis of the nails.**

A   Psoriatic arthritis is one of the seronegative spondyloarthritides. It is
important to remember that the skin manifestations may occur subsequent to joint involvement. The patient in the question shows a typical
presentation of DIP joint involvement with signs of nail dystrophy.
Radiologically, the affective joints show central erosion rather than the
juxta-articular involvement that is seen in rheumatoid arthritis.
About 5 per cent of patients with psoriasis may present with marked
deformity in the fingers caused by severe periarticular osteolysis. This is
known as arthritis mutilans.

43 Joint pain

Answers: L F K J D

**A 64-year-old patient who has recently been started on medication
for hypertension presents with a very painful, hot, swollen metatarsophalangeal joint.**

L   Gout is associated with hyperuricaemia and therefore acute attacks may
be precipitated by impaired excretion/increased production of uric acid.
Drugs that impair the excretion of uric acid include thiazide diuretics and
aspirin. States of increased cell turnover and thus increased purine
turnover, e.g. myelo-/lymphoproliferative states or carcinoma, can predispose to gout. Obesity, diabetes mellitus, high alcohol intake and
hypertension are associated with hyperuricaemia.

**A 12-year-old haemophiliac presents to A&E with severe pain after
falling over and banging his right knee.**

F   Bleeding into the joint (haemarthrosis) may occur in all patients but is
more common in those with acquired/inherited disorders of coagulation
such as haemophilia.

**A 55-year-old man presents to A&E with fever and an exquisitely
painful right knee. On examination his right knee is red, hot and
swollen. Purulent fluid is aspirated from the joint.**

K   The differential diagnosis of a monoarthritis is septic arthritis,
osteoarthritis, crystal-induced arthritis, or trauma-related or a single
joint manifestation of a multi-joint disease.

Septic arthritis is a medical emergency and so, when a patient presents with a red, hot, swollen knee, treatment for any other possible diagnosis must not be initiated before septic arthritis is excluded. The joint space should be aspirated and the fluid sent for urgent Gram staining and culture as soon as possible.

A 60-year-old woman presents with a painful swollen knee. Her radiograph shows chondrocalcinosis and joint aspiration reveals presence of weakly positive birefringent crystals.

J Pseudogout refers to the acute synovitis caused by the deposition of calcium pyrophosphate crystals into a joint. The knee and the wrist are the two most commonly affected sites. Diagnosis is made by detection of crystals that are weakly positively birefringent in plane polarized light. Risk factors include hypovolaemia, hyperparathyroidism, diabetes, haemochromatosis, acromegaly and any other pre-existing arthritis.

A 65-year-old woman presents with a 1-month history of pain and stiffness in her shoulders, worse in the mornings. She says that she was treated in hospital last year for headache and jaw pain.

D Polymyalgia rheumatica is associated with giant cell arteritis and is very rare before the age of 50 years. Patients also often complain of fatigue and depression. It is often associated with a high erythrocyte sedimentation rate (ESR). Oral prednisolone is the treatment of choice.

44 Pain in the hip

Answers: A M C J E

An obese 12-year-old boy presents with pain in his right hip. On examination the hip is flexed, abducted and externally rotated. His mother has suffered from TB in the past.

A This is a classic presentation of slipped femoral epiphysis and the previous history of TB in the mother is not significant. The patient is often obese and presents with limping and pain in the groin, thigh or knee. This condition is most common in the 10- to 16-year age group. A lateral radiograph is required to show the abnormality.
Tuberculous arthritis is very rare in the UK, affecting mostly elderly people and infants.

A 6-year-old boy presents with a pain in the hip and a limp. All movements at the hip are limited. His radiograph shows decrease in size of the nuclear femoral head with patchy density.

M Perthes' disease is osteochondritis of the femoral head and classically affects children in a younger age group compared with slipped femoral epiphysis (around 3–11 years). It is around four times more common in males. The younger the patient on presentation, the better the prognosis. In many cases, rest is sufficient treatment. In severe disease, surgery may be indicated.

A 3-year-old girl presents to the orthopaedic clinic with a waddling gait. Her mother says that there has been a delay in walking. On examination there is an extra crease on the left thigh.

C Congenital dislocation of the hip (CDH) is around six times more common in females and is more common after breech delivery. Ortolani's test and the Barlow manoeuvre are performed to identify this condition, which is bilateral in about a third of cases. In Ortolani's test the examiner holds the baby's thighs with the thumbs placed medially and the fingers resting on the greater trochanters. The examiner flexes the hips to 90° and gently abducts to almost 90°. In CDH this movement is difficult and, if pressure is applied to the greater trochanter, there is an audible click as the dislocation reduces. Barlow's test involves the examiner grasping the upper thigh with the thumb placed in the groin and attempting to lever the femoral head in and out of the acetabulum as he or she abducts and adducts the thigh.

An 80-year-old woman presents to A&E after a fall. On examination the left hip is adducted, externally rotated and excruciatingly painful.

J Remember that the hip is adducted, externally rotated and shortened after a fractured neck of femur.

An 8-year-old boy presents to A&E with marked limping and pain in the right hip, which resolves within 48 h. His radiographs show no abnormality at the hip or other joint involvement. Bone scan 2 weeks later is also normal. The patient's mother suffers from osteoarthritis.

E The patient must have a normal radiograph for the diagnosis to be made. This condition is also known as 'irritable hip.' Transient synovitis is a diagnosis of exclusion, i.e. the diagnosis is made only when all other possible diagnoses have been eliminated.

45 Back pain

Answers: K G J C D

A 22-year-old man complains of stiffness in the lower back and buttock pain that is relieved by exercise. He also suffers from bouts of painful red eye. His ESR is raised. His radiograph shows blurring of the upper vertebral rims of the lumbar spine.

K Buttock pain is caused by sacroiliitis. Blurring of the vertebral rims is an early sign on a radiograph resulting from enthesitis at the insertion of intervertebral ligaments. Later, persistent enthesitis leads to the formation of bony spurs called syndesmophytes.

A 60-year-old woman presents with constant backache. Her ESR and serum calcium are markedly elevated.

G   Back pain is common in older people and the cause is often benign. However, constant symptoms, raised ESR and raised serum calcium raise the suspicion of underlying myeloma.

A 65-year-old man with osteoarthritis complains of back pain worse on walking along, with aching and heaviness in both legs that force him to stop walking. Pain is relieved slowly after rest or leaning forward.

J   This is a classic description of spinal claudication (leaning forward opens the spinal canal and relieves pain). In vascular claudication the pain is quickly relieved on rest, whereas the relief from pain occurs later in spinal claudication. Operative decompression can be very successful in treating symptoms of pain in patients who are severely affected.

A 13-year-old girl complains of backache and fatigue. She is worried that she is becoming increasingly round-shouldered. On examination, she has a smooth thoracic kyphosis. Her radiograph shows wedge-shaped vertebral bodies in the thoracic spine.

C   Scheuermann's disease is a rare condition that typically affects females during puberty. There is abnormal ossification of ring epiphyses of thoracic vertebrae. The deforming forces are greatest at the anterior border of the vertebrae giving rise to the described wedge-shaped vertebral bodies (i.e. narrower anteriorly). Management depends on the degree of kyphosis and ranges from back-strengthening exercises and postural training in those mildly affected to operative correction and fusion in those with severe kyphosis.

A 35-year-old tourist complains of severe back pain with inability to straighten up after lifting a suitcase yesterday. He now presents with weakness of his big toe extension and loss of sensation on the outer side of the calf.

D   He is showing symptoms of compression at the L5 level.

46 Rheumatological conditions

Answers: H A B K D

A 45-year-old woman complains of cold numb fingers and difficulty in swallowing. On examination she has tight skin, thickening of the fingers and telangiectasia.

H   Systemic sclerosis is a multisystem connective tissue disease that is classified as either limited or diffuse cutaneous scleroderma.
Limited cutaneous scleroderma is the milder form and usually starts with Raynaud's phenomenon followed by skin changes. The characteristic

tight skin gives rise to the 'beak' nose and small mouth aperture (microstomia). Limited scleroderma is associated with the presence of anti-centromere antibodies. The term 'CREST syndrome' was the previous name for limited cutaneous scleroderma because it summarized the signs of calcinosis, Raynaud's phenomenon, oesophageal dysmotility, sclerodactyly and telangiectasia that can be found in affected patients. Diffuse scleroderma is characterized by oedema and extensive sclerosis which can involve most of the body including major organs, e.g. heart, lungs, kidneys. Diffuse scleroderma is associated with the presence of anti-topoisomerase and anti-RNA antibodies.

A 51-year-old woman complains of weakness in her shoulders and thighs. She has a significantly raised CK level.

A   Polymyositis is an autoimmune condition characterized by a non-suppurative inflammation of striated muscle that gives rise to a symmetrical proximal myopathy. Unlike other causes of pain and weakness (e.g. polymyalgia rheumatica) CK is characteristically elevated. Electromyography (EMG) shows fibrillation potentials in this condition.

Dermatomyositis describes polymyositis associated with a heliotrope (purple) rash on the cheeks and other areas of skin exposed to sunlight. Dermatomyositis is associated with an increased risk of malignancy. Treatment is with steroids and other immunosuppressive agents.

A 25-year-old man has been referred to rheumatology clinic with multiple painful stiff joints and uveitis. He also complains of ulcers on his penis and mouth.

B   Behçet's disease is an inflammatory disorder of unknown aetiology characterized by signs of orogenital ulceration and eye lesions, e.g. uveitis, retinal vein occlusion. A positive skin pathergy test is pathognomonic. A positive result involves the development of a pustule on the skin within 24 h of being pricked at that exact point with a sterile needle.

Erythema nodosum is a recognized cutaneous manifestation of Behçet's disease.

Neurological manifestations of Behçet's disease include meningo-encephalitis, dementia and cerebral vein occlusion.

Behçet's disease is managed with immunosuppressants, e.g. cortico-steroids, ciclosporin.

A 45-year-old woman presents with dryness in the eyes and mouth. Her Schirmer's test is positive.

K   Primary Sjögren's syndrome (SS) is characterized by symptoms of dry eyes (xerophthalmia) and dry mouth (xerostomia). Secondary SS describes the above symptoms in the presence of other autoimmune disease processes, e.g. rheumatoid arthritis.

Anti-ro antibodies are found in 75 per cent of patients with primary SS but only 10–15 per cent patients with secondary SS.
A Schirmer's test can be used to identify insufficient production of tears. The test involves placing a strip of filter paper on the inside of the lower lid. A wetting (measured by the distance the water is absorbed up the paper) of less than 10 mm in 5 min implies defective tear production. Salivary gland biopsy to identify the focal infiltrate of lymphocytes is the best single test for diagnosis.
Management involves treating the symptoms with artificial tears and saliva.

A patient presents to rheumatology clinic with recurrent attacks of pain and swelling in the nose and external ear.

D   Polychondritis is an inflammatory condition affecting cartilage that mainly affects the nose and the ear. Other features include vasculitis and seronegative arthritis.

47 Complications of fractures

Answers: A H E G L

A 25-year-old man presents with a blue right arm with absent radial pulse and painful passive finger extension after a supracondylar fracture of humerus.

A   Fracture can lead to ischaemia in the distal limb by direct injury to the blood vessel or by the effect of oedema increasing the pressure within the osteofascial compartment, which limits perfusion. In compartment syndrome, the increased pressure can lead to profound ischaemia with necrosis of muscle and nerve tissue. This is a surgical emergency requiring prompt decompression by open fasciotomy. Once muscle tissue has become infarcted, it is replaced by inelastic fibrous tissue giving rise to the complication of Volkmann's ischaemic contracture.

A 40-year-old woman presents 5 weeks after a radial fracture with a painful swollen hand. The hand is cold and cyanosed with heightened temperature sensitivity.

H   This condition is now known as complex regional pain syndrome type 1. The pain and swelling are close to, but not exactly at, the area of injury. The skin may be oedematous and there may be altered sweat production. Its aetiology is unknown.

A 70-year-old woman complains of right-sided pleuritic chest pain 10 days after a fractured neck of femur.

E   Pleuritic chest pain after orthopaedic/pelvic surgery should invoke strong suspicion of pulmonary embolus.

A 60-year-old woman complains of pain, swelling and reduced mobility 4 months after suffering a fractured neck of femur. Her radiograph shows absence of callus at fracture site.

G   Absence of callus at the fracture site implies delayed union. Malunion is diagnosed only if the radiograph shows that the medullary cavity has been closed off.

A 65-year-old woman who falls on an outstretched arm shows weakness of wrist extensors.

L   Radial nerve supplies motor innervation to the extensors of the wrist. Look out for signs of radial nerve injury after fracture/dislocation of the elbow, fracture of the humerus and injury to the axillary region.

48 Management of fractures

Answers: J E F B H

A 24-year-old man presents with a swollen painful hand after a falling over playing squash. His radiograph reveals a scaphoid fracture.

J   The wrist is held in dorsiflexion. A plaster cast from the wrist to above the knuckle provides insufficient support.

A 1-year-old baby requires traction after fracture of the right femur.

E   This means of traction is suitable up to the age of 2 years.

A 65-year-old woman requires treatment for displaced fractured neck of femur.

F   This is the management of choice and mobilization can begin immediately because internal fixation holds a fracture very securely.

A 35-year-old woman presents after a fall on an outstretched arm. Her radiograph shows an undisplaced transverse fracture of the right humerus.

B   A collar-and-cuff sling provides sufficient support for this fracture. A broad sling is used to stabilize a fractured clavicle.

A 75-year-old woman suffers a displaced Colles' fracture.

H   The cast is applied from just below the elbow to the palm of the hand with the wrist in the neutral position/slightly flexed.

49 Fall on the outstretched hand

Answers: F A J E K

A 24-year-old woman presents with pain on wrist movements after a fall on to her hand. On examination there is tenderness and swelling in the anatomical snuffbox.

F   The anatomical snuffbox (ASB) is a triangular depression best seen when the thumb is extended. It is bounded anteriorly by the tendons abductor pollicis longus and extensor pollicis brevis, and posteriorly by the tendon of the extensor pollicis longus. The scaphoid and trapezium lie at the base of the ASB. The radial styloid process and the base of the first metacarpal can be felt proximally and distally to the floor respectively. The radial artery and a superficial branch of the radial nerve cross the ASB.

Pain and swelling at the ASB after injury to the arm/hand suggest fracture of the scaphoid.

If there is high clinical suspicion of fractured scaphoid, but no positive radiological findings, a plaster cast may be applied and a radiograph repeated 2 weeks later (the fracture may become more clear on the radiograph later).

A 68-year-old woman presents with fracture at distal radial head with dorsal displacement of distal fragment after a fall.

A   A displaced Colles' fracture is sometimes described as exhibiting a 'dinner-fork' deformity. This injury is more common in older women where osteoporosis has increased the susceptibility to fracture. A Smith's fracture is a form of 'reverse' Colles' fracture where the radial fragment is angled forwards. These fractures are rare and often unstable, requiring internal fixation.

A 7-year-old boy presents with a swollen painful elbow after a fall. He is unable to move the arm because of the pain.

J   This injury is more common in children after a fall on the outstretched hand. It is imperative to look for any signs of damage to the brachial artery. The elbow should be kept extended to avoid arterial damage. Displaced fractures are surgical emergencies and treated by reduction under general anaesthesia.

A 19-year-old rugby player falls on a backward stretched hand and presents with loss of shoulder contour and absent sensation on a patch below the shoulder.

E   The loss of sensation results from damage to the axillary nerve. On a radiograph the humeral head lies anterior and inferior to the glenoid. The shoulder can be reduced with the Kocher's manoeuvre. The elbow is flexed to 90° and traction applied. The arm is slowly externally rotated to about 90°, brought across the chest and then finally internally rotated.

A 40-year-old woman presents after a fall on an outstretched hand with wrist drop.

K   The radial nerve is susceptible to injury with fracture of the humeral shaft as it winds around the humerus in the spiral groove.

50 Shoulder problems

Answers: G E A K D

A 21-year-old woman presents with a very painful shoulder locked in medial rotation after an epileptic fit.

G   On examination the coracoid process may be prominent and the humeral head felt posteriorly. A lateral film is essential to spot the posterior sub-luxation. An epileptic seizure is a common cause of posterior dislocation of the shoulder.

A 55-year-old man complains of shoulder pain aggravated in abduction of arm between 60° and 120°.

E   This patient is describing a painful arc syndrome. The pain of supraspina-tus tendonitis can be elicited if the examiner elevates an internally rotated arm causing the supraspinatus tendon to be impinged against the anterior inferior acromion. This pain is reduced/alleviated if the test is repeated after injecting local anaesthetic into the subacromial space.
Treatment includes the use of physiotherapy and patient education with respect to particular arm movements/activities. Corticosteroid/local anaesthetic injections are useful in the acute setting.

A 30-year-old bodybuilder presents with an aching shoulder. Flexing elbow reveals a prominent lump in the upper arm.

A   This injury occurs after lifting/pulling activity. Good function usually returns and surgery is rarely indicated.

A 50-year-old man complains of a 9-month history of stiffness in the shoulder. The shoulder was originally extremely painful but now only the stiffness remains.

K   Adhesive capsulitis is more commonly known as 'frozen shoulder.' Examination should reveal marked reduction in passive and active movement. There may be some history of previous injury reported but this is not always present. There is no definitive treatment but NSAIDs, intra-articular steroids and physiotherapy can reduce pain and increase the range of movement in some patients.

A 65-year-old woman presents with shoulder pain and restricted movement in all directions. Her radiograph shows reduced joint space and subchondral sclerosis.

D   Reduced joint space, subchondral sclerosis, subchondral cysts and osteo-phytes are features suggestive of osteoarthritis.

51 Knee problems

Answers: F J A L E

> A 22-year-old figure-skater presents with a painful locked knee with limited extension after a twisting injury.

F   Meniscal tears usually result from a twisting injury. The displaced torn portion can become jammed between the femur and tibia, resulting in locking.

> A 24-year-old footballer presents with a painful knee after a tackle from behind. With the quadriceps relaxed, the anterior glide of the tibia on the femur is 1.0 cm.

J   With the knee flexed at 90°, anterior glide of the tibia on the femur should be only about 0.5 cm. Excessive glide anteriorly implies anterior cruciate ligament damage; excessive glide posteriorly implies posterior cruciate ligament damage.

> A 14-year-old girl successfully treated for rickets 3 years ago shows bow-legged deformity.

A   In valgus deformity the distal part is lateral to the midline.

> A 16-year-old boy complains of a painful knee after exercise and a tender lump over the tibial tuberosity.

L   Osgood–Schlatter disease is more common in older children. Pain is felt particularly on straight leg raise against resistance. The presence of a lump over the tibial tuberosity is diagnostic. Spontaneous recovery is usual but it is advisable to avoid sport during this time.

> A 50-year-old carpet layer presents with a swelling directly over the patella. The joint is normal.

E   Pre-patellar bursitis is also known as housemaid's knee. The condition is usually treated by the use of firm bandaging and by abstaining from the kneeling position that has caused the injury.

52 Management of painful joints

Answers: A H B C G

> A 24-year-old man presented with lower back pain and stiffness that was worse in the morning. He has a question-mark posture.

A   This is a presentation of ankylosing spondylitis. Patients often report improvement of stiffness with hydrotherapy. Exercise is preferred to rest for the improvement of back symptoms.

An 80-year-old man with a 30-year history of rheumatoid arthritis presents to A&E with fever and pain in the right knee. On examination his right knee is red, hot and swollen. Aspirated synovial fluid is frankly purulent.

H   Aspiration of the joint and culture is required to establish whether the acutely swollen knee has resulted from inflammation, infection or a crystal arthropathy. Intravenous flucloxacillin plus benzylpenicillin is also a popular drug combination that is used until sensitivities have been established.

A 65-year-old woman recently diagnosed with osteoarthritis requires medication for joint pain.

B   Paracetamol should be prescribed before NSAIDs for relief of osteoarthritic pain. The use of NSAIDs for analgesia can be problematic in a chronic condition such as osteoarthritis as a result of the risk of gastrointestinal bleeding with long-term use.

A 64-year-old woman who has been successfully treated for acute gout requires prophylactic medication.

C   Colchicine is an alternative to NSAIDs in an acute presentation of gout in patients in whom NSAIDs are contraindicated, e.g. those with allergy or heart failure. Allopurinol is a xanthine oxidase inhibitor that decreases the production of uric acid and is used only for prophylaxis. It should not be used in treatment of acute gout and, in fact, its use may actually provoke acute gout during that period.

A 65-year-old woman with polymyalgia rheumatica.

G   Oral prednisolone is the treatment of choice for polymyalgia rheumatica.

53 Disease-modifying anti-rheumatic drugs (DMARDs)

Answers: H B C K E

CT of patient on long-term DMARD treatment shows pulmonary and hepatic fibrosis.

H   Methotrexate is also indicated in the treatment of malignant disease and severe psoriasis unresponsive to conventional therapy. Methotrexate can show cumulative toxicity and so renal and liver function tests should be carried out every 2–3 months while on treatment (monitor weekly until therapy is stabilized). Other examples of drugs causing pulmonary fibrosis are bleomycin, amiodarone and nitrofurantoin.

Fertility testing reveals oligospermia in a 48-year-old man on DMARD treatment.

B   Sulfasalazine (sulphasalazine) is known to cause a reversible oligospermia in up to 70 per cent of males treated for over 3 years.

A patient complains of grossly swollen gums.

C Monitoring kidney function is important as a result of the adverse effects of nephrotoxicity and hyperkalaemia. Note that a dose-dependent increase in serum urea and creatinine is seen during the first few weeks of treatment.
Gum hypertrophy is also a recognized adverse effect of phenytoin and calcium channel blockers.

A patient taking an intramuscular DMARD presents with an itchy erythematous rash covering the whole body.

K Exfoliative dermatitis is a medical emergency. Such a widespread inflammation of the skin can have severe complications, including hypothermia, fluid loss, hypoalbuminaemia and 'capillary leak syndrome' (inflammatory cytokine cascade mediates vascular leakage and oedema in major organs). Sulphonamides can also give rise to this presentation in some individuals.

A 65-year-old woman patient presents with gross irreversible retinopathy.

E Retinopathy associated with hydroxychloroquine is irreversible and so regular ophthalmological monitoring is required.

REVISION BOXES

Orthopaedics and rheumatology

Seronegative refers to the fact that the conditions are not associated with production of rheumatoid factor. These conditions commonly appear in EMQs (Box 1). You should particularly look out for the associations mentioned as they may appear as clues in the EMQ.

Box 1 Seronegative spondyloarthritides

Seronegative factors	Condition
• Triad of urethritis, conjunctivitis, arthritis Associated lesions include circinate balanitis Keratoderma blenorrhagica Mouth ulcers	Reiter's syndrome [42]
• Young male, buttock/sacroiliac pain worse in morning, relieved by exercise; syndesmophytes, 'bamboo spine' on radiograph Associations include 4As: arthritis, anterior uveitis, apical lung fibrosis, aortic regurgitation	Ankylosing spondylitis [45, 52]
• Nail dystrophy, 'pitting' Joints show central erosion on radiograph Can be highly deforming (arthritis mutilans)	Psoriatic arthritis [42]
• Arthritis in ulcerative colitis (UC)/Crohn's disease patient Asymmetrical, mainly affects lower limbs	Enteropathic arthropathy

Box 2 summarizes the distinctive features of some connective tissue diseases that may assist you in answering EMQS.

Box 2 Connective tissue disease

Feature	CT disease
• Usually woman: persistently cold, cyanosed fingers	Raynaud's phenomenon
Calcinosis (nodules)	Systemic sclerosis [46]
Raynaud's phenomenon (in almost all cases)	
Oesophageal dysmotility (difficulty swallowing)	
Sclerodactyly	
Telangiectasia	
• More common in Turkish, Iranian patients	Behçet's disease [46]
Orogenital ulceration, uveitis, arthritis	
Pathergy reaction is pathognomonic	
• Proximal muscle weakness, pain and tenderness	Polymyositis [31, 46]
↑serum CK (creatine kinase)	
Above plus heliotrope (purple) rash	Dermatomyositis [46]
• Dry eyes, dry mouth	Sjögren's syndrome [46]
Positive Schirmer's test	

Vasculitis can give rise to pathology in several organs and must therefore be considered in the differential diagnosis of a patient with an unidentified multi-system disorder.

Box 3 summarizes some of the vasculitides with distinctive features that commonly appear in EMQs.

Box 3 Vasculitides

Feature	Vasculitide
• Usually elderly patient with headache Scalp tenderness, jaw claudication very suggestive Amaurosis fugax, sudden unilateral blindness can occur associated with polymyalgia rheumatica	Temporal/giant cell arteritis [29, 40]
• Granulomas in respiratory tract, generalized vasculitis Classic anti-neutrophil cytoplasmic antibody (cANCA), anti-PR3 positive	Wegener's granulomatosis [13]
• Usually child (particularly under age 5) Purpuric rash over buttocks, extensor surfaces Associated with arthritis, abdominal pain, nephritis	Henoch–Schönlein purpura [69]

continued overleaf

continued
- Usually middle-aged male   Churg–Strauss syndrome
  Asthma, rhinitis and systemic vasculitis
  +++ eosinophilia
- Usually under 5 years: Kawasaki's disease
  Main features are:
  – protracted fever (over 5 days)
  – acute cervical lymphadenopathy
  – bilateral non-purulent conjunctivitis
  – dry, cracked, fissured lips
  – redness, oedema of palms and soles
  Platelets, CRP (C-reactive protein) usually ↑↑

In examination EMQs certain autoantibodies tend to be associated with particular diseases.

Sensitivity refers to the proportion of patients with a disease that have a positive result. Therefore an autoantibody test with high sensitivity is useful for screening purposes.

Specificity refers to the proportion of patients without the disease who have a negative test result. Therefore a specific autoantibody test with high specificity is useful for confirming diagnosis but not general screening.

Autoantibodies with high specificity are often mentioned in EMQs to aid diagnosis (Box 4).

Box 4 Antibodies and screening

Antibody	Diagnosis
Anti double-stranded DNA	SLE (systemic lupus erythematosus)
Anti-Jo1 antibodies	Polymyositis
Anti-centromere	Limited systemic sclerosis
Anti-topoisomerase	Diffuse systemic sclerosis
cANCA, anti-PR3	Wegener's granulomatosis
α-Endomysial antibody	Coeliac disease

Box 5 summarizes some typical presenting symptoms/signs that you may find in an EMQ that is describing a particular problem in the upper limb.

Box 5 Orthopaedic presentations: upper limb

Presentation	Problem
• Painful shoulder following seizure	Posterior dislocation shoulder [50]
• Failure to abduct shoulder after dislocation	Axillary nerve injury [49]

continued overleaf

continued

• Winged scapula	Long thoracic nerve injury [32]
'Dinner fork' deformity	Colles' fracture [49]
• Forced adduction and flexion thumb elicits pain on radial side wrist	De Quervain's syndrome
• Thickening, fibrosis palmar fascia	Dupuytren's contracture
• Pain, paraesthesia median nerve distribution	Carpal tunnel syndrome

Box 6 summarizes some typical presenting symptoms/signs that you may find in an EMQ that is describing a particular problem in the lower limb.

Box 6 Orthopaedic presentations: lower limb

Presentation	Problem
Flexed, adducted and externally rotated leg	Femoral shaft fracture
Locked knee, positive McMurray's test	Meniscal tear [51]
Drop foot after hip replacement	Sciatic nerve injury [36]
Drop foot after knee injury	Common peroneal nerve injury [32]
Excessive anterior glide tibia on femur	Anterior cruciate ligament injury [51]
Excessive posterior glide tibia on femur	Posterior cruciate ligament injury
Prominent tender tibial tubercle	Osgood–Schlatter disease [51]

Radiological findings can often prove to be the best clue to the correct answer in an EMQ.

Box 7 summarizes some radiological findings that are typical of particular conditions.

Box 7 Radiological findings

Findings	Condition
• Loss of joint space Subchondral sclerosis Subchondral cysts Osteophytes	Osteoarthritis [42]
• Loss of joint space Juxta-articular osteoporosis Erosions, subluxation joints	Rheumatoid arthritis [42, 53]
• Localized enlargement of bone with deformity (e.g. enlarged skull, bowed tibia)	Paget's disease
• Syndesmophytes 'Bamboo-spine' appearance	Ankylosing spondylitis [45, 52]
• 'Sunray' spiculation	Osteosarcoma
• 'Onion-peel sign'	Ewing's sarcoma

SECTION 6: THE ABDOMEN AND SURGERY

QUESTIONS

54 Abdominal pain

A	large bowel obstruction	H	aortic dissection
B	acute pancreatitis	I	diverticulosis
C	perforated viscus	J	duodenal ulcer
D	appendicitis	K	renal colic
E	small bowel obstruction	L	colorectal carcinoma
F	acute cholecystitis	M	mesenteric adenitis
G	ulcerative colitis			

For each clinical scenario below, give the most likely cause for the clinical findings. Each option may be used only once.

1   A 45-year-old man with a history of gallstones presents in A&E with severe epigastric pain radiating to the back and vomiting.

2   A 28-year-old man presents with sharp left loin and left upper quadrant pain radiating to the groin. He is not jaundiced.

3   A 44-year-old woman presents with continuous right upper quadrant pain, vomiting and fever. Murphy's sign is positive.

4   A 26-year-old man with a previous history of abdominal surgery presents with colicky central abdominal pain, rapidly followed by production of copious bile-stained vomitus.

5   A 50-year-old man presents with epigastric pain worse at night and relieved by eating or drinking milk.

Answers: see page 166.

55 Abdominal pain

A	hepatitis	H	Crohn's disease
B	irritable bowel syndrome	I	primary biliary cirrhosis
C	umbilical hernia	J	carcinoma of sigmoid colon
D	primary sclerosing cholangitis	K	acute appendicitis
E	perforated duodenal ulcer	L	gastric ulcer
F	small bowel obstruction	M	pneumothorax
G	ulcerative colitis			

For each clinical scenario below, give the most likely cause for the clinical findings. Each option may be used only once.

1   A 21-year-old student presents with a cramping diffuse abdominal pain associated with alternating constipation and diarrhoea. Investigations are normal.

2   A 55-year-old smoker presents with severe epigastric pain. The chest radiograph reveals air under the diaphragm.

3   A 9-year-old girl presents with fever, nausea and right iliac fossa pain. She says that the pain 'was around my belly-button before'.

4   A 35-year-old man presents with weight loss, diarrhoea and abdominal pain. On examination, he has aphthous ulcers in the mouth and a mass is palpable in the right iliac fossa. Blood tests reveal low serum vitamin B_{12} and folate.

5   A 45-year-old woman on treatment for TB presents with abdominal pain and malaise. On examination she is jaundiced.

Answers: see page 167.

56 Abdominal masses

A	renal cell carcinoma	G	diverticulosis
B	ovarian carcinoma	H	hepatocellular carcinoma
C	gastric carcinoma	I	caecal carcinoma
D	sigmoid carcinoma	J	psoas abscess
E	fibroids	K	abdominal aortic aneurysm
F	pancreatic pseudocyst	L	ovarian cyst

For each clinical scenario below, give the most likely cause for the clinical findings. Each option may be used only once.

1   A 65-year-old man collapses in the street. On examination he has an umbilical mass that is expansile and pulsatile.

2   A 75-year-old man with a 3-month history of dyspepsia presents with weight loss and abdominal distension. On examination a 3.5 cm, hard, irregular, tender epigastric mass can be felt which moves on respiration. Percussion of the distended abdomen reveals shifting dullness. The left supraclavicular node is palpable.

3   A 70-year-old woman presents with a mass in the right iliac fossa and severe microcytic anaemia. On examination the mass is firm, irregular and 4 cm in diameter. The lower edge is palpable.

4   A 35-year-old woman is worried about an abdominal mass that has grown over the last 6 months and a similar length history of very heavy menstrual bleeding with no intermenstrual bleeding. On examination a knobbly mass can be felt in the middle lower quadrant that is dull to percussion. The lower edge is not palpable. She is otherwise well.

5   A 70 year old with alcohol problems presents with a tender upper abdominal mass. Computed tomography (CT) shows a thick-walled, rounded, fluid-filled mass adjacent to the pancreas.

Answers: see page 168.

57 Liver diseases

A	hepatocellular carcinoma	G	fulminant liver failure
B	hepatic encephalopathy	H	Wilson's disease
C	liver metastasis	I	hepatic haemangioma
D	α_1-antitrypsin deficiency	J	primary biliary cirrhosis
E	alcoholic cirrhosis	K	haemochromatosis
F	acute viral hepatitis E	L	acute viral hepatitis B

For each clinical scenario below, give the most likely cause for the clinical findings. Each option may be used once only.

1   A 69-year-old retired bricklayer presents with weight loss, fever and right upper quadrant pain. On examination, a hard, irregular liver can be felt on palpation. Serum AFP is grossly elevated.

2   A 45-year-old man presents with arthralgia, tiredness and development of diabetes. On examination his skin is pigmented and blood tests show increased serum ferritin.

3   A 60-year-old publican presents with signs of spider naevi, gynaecomastia and testicular atrophy. His hands show clubbing and leukonychia.

4   A 20-year-old man with a history of liver problems in the past presents with tremor and dysarthria with developing dyskinesias. Slit-lamp examination reveals a greenish-brown ring at the corneoscleral junction.

5   A 50-year-old man presents with signs of chronic liver disease with a history of early onset pulmonary emphysema. He is a non-smoker and is teetotal. His father had a similar history.

Answers: see page 169.

58 Causes of splenomegaly

A	malaria	G	Weil's disease
B	pernicious anaemia	H	infectious mononucleosis
C	sarcoidosis	I	cutaneous leishmaniasis
D	idiopathic thrombocytopenic purpura	J	Budd–Chiari syndrome
		K	myeloma
E	Gaucher's disease	L	Felty's syndrome
F	infective endocarditis	M	acute lymphoblastic leukaemia

For each clinical scenario below, give the most likely cause for the clinical findings. Each option may be used only once.

1 A 75-year-old woman with long-standing rheumatoid arthritis is seen to have splenomegaly on abdominal examination. Her full blood count shows anaemia and a low white cell count.

2 A 35-year-old man presents with an insidious onset of hepatosplenomegaly with marked pigmentation on the forehead and hands. He is anaemic and has a history of pathological fractures.

3 A 23-year-old man presents with a week's history of fever and sore throat. He developed a macular rash after being prescribed ampicillin by his GP. On examination he has enlarged posterior cervical nodes, palatal petechiae and splenomegaly.

4 A 21-year-old female backpacker returning from India presents with flu-like symptoms followed by a periodic fever. She is anaemic, jaundiced and has moderate splenomegaly.

5 A 28-year-old woman presents with abdominal pain, vomiting and jaundice. On examination she has tender hepatomegaly and ascites. She has a history of recurrent miscarriages.

Answers: see page 171.

59 Jaundice

A	autoimmune hepatitis	H	Wilson's disease
B	hepatitis C	I	haemochromatosis
C	hepatitis A	J	Gilbert's syndrome
D	iatrogenic hepatitis	K	Dubin–Johnson syndrome
E	rotor syndrome	L	haemolytic anaemia
F	primary biliary cirrhosis	M	primary sclerosing cholangitis
G	hepatocellular carcinoma		

For each clinical scenario below, give the most likely cause for the clinical findings. Each option may be used only once.

1   A 24 year old presents with nausea, malaise and jaundice. He returned 3 weeks ago from a holiday abroad. On examination he has a moderate hepatosplenomegaly and tender cervical lymphadenopathy. He has dark urine and pale stools.

2   A 35-year-old woman presents with fever, malaise and jaundice. On examination she has moderate hepatomegaly. She is anti-smooth muscle antibody and anti-nuclear antibody positive.

3   A 25-year-old man presents with recurrent episodes of asymptomatic jaundice.

4   A 4-year-old patient presents with anaemia and mild jaundice. Hb 7 g/dl, reticulocytes 14 per cent. Electrophoresis result pending.

5   A 45-year-old man with ulcerative colitis presents with jaundice, pruritus and abdominal pain. Alkaline phosphatase (ALP) is raised and anti-mitochondrial antibodies negative.

Answers: see page 172.

60 Breast conditions

A   Paget's disease
B   phyllodes tumour
C   mammary haemangioma
D   galactocele
E   chronic breast abscess
F   metastatic carcinoma of breast
G   benign eczema of nipple

H   fibroadenoma
I   postpartum fat necrosis
J   gynaecomastia
K   mastitis
L   dermatitis herpetiformis
M   duct ectasia

For each clinical scenario below, give the most likely cause for the clinical findings. Each option may be used only once.

1   A 75-year-old woman presents to her GP with a breast lump in the upper outer quadrant. On examination the lump is hard and irregular. There is axillary lymphadenopathy.

2   A 53-year-old woman presents with nipple retraction and a greeny-yellow discharge. Her ductogram shows dilated breast ducts.

3   A 21-year-old woman presents with a smooth, non-tender, highly mobile mass on the upper outer quadrant of the right breast. Fine needle aspiration does not reveal malignant features.

4   A 70-year-old woman presents with a worsening eczema-like rash overlying the areola and nipple. The rash does not itch. On examination a palpable mass can be felt under the rash.

5   A 26-year-old woman presents a fortnight post partum with a painful, enlarged left breast. On examination she is pyrexial and her breast is tender and inflamed. There are no palpable masses.

Answers: see page 174.

61 Presentation with a lump

A	histiocytoma	H	neurofibroma
B	myosarcoma	I	sebaceous cyst
C	ganglion	J	keloid
D	abscess	K	Marjolin's ulcer
E	lipoma	L	keratoacanthoma
F	carbuncle	M	osteoma
G	furuncle		

For each description of a lump(s) below, give the most likely cause for the clinical findings. Each option may be used only once.

1 A 22-year-old man presents with a lump on the scalp. Examination reveals a smooth, spherical, tense lump. A small punctum can be seen on the surface.

2 A 33-year-old man presents with a swelling on the upper arm that has been growing slowly for a number of years. Examination reveals a soft, compressible, non-tender, lobulated mass.

3 A 28-year-old man presents with a painless swelling on the dorsum of the right hand. Examination reveals a smooth, spherical, tense, 1.5 cm swelling. The over-lying skin can be drawn over it.

4 A 29-year-old man presents with two mobile fusiform-shaped lumps on the forearm. Each swelling feels like firm rubber and causes tingling in the hand on pressure.

5 A 65-year-old woman presents with a rapidly growing lump just below the eye. Examination reveals a 2 cm smooth, round, skin-coloured lump with a black central core. The lump is freely mobile over subcutaneous tissues.

Answers: see page 175.

62 Lumps in the neck

A	branchial cyst	H	sternomastoid tumour
B	pharyngeal pouch	I	carotid body tumour
C	tuberculous abscess	J	subclavian aneurysm
D	toxic goitre	K	cervical rib
E	thyroglossal cyst	L	tonsillar node
F	sebaceous cyst	M	anaplastic carcinoma
G	cystic hygroma			

For each clinical scenario below, give the most likely cause for the clinical findings. Each option may be used only once.

1   A 28-year-old man presents with halitosis and regurgitation of food. He has a lump in the posterior triangle.

2   A 20-year-old woman presents with a small painless midline swelling that has increased in size. The swelling moves upwards on protruding the tongue.

3   An 8-year-old girl presents with a painful lump just below the angle of the jaw. She has a sore throat and is pyrexial.

4   A 22-year-old man presents with a lump behind the anterior border of sternocleidomastoid on the upper left side of the neck. He has had the lump for a number of years but it has recently become painful.

5   A parent brings a 4-year-old boy to clinic with a large swelling at the base of the posterior triangle. The swelling is soft and fluctuant and transilluminates brilliantly.

Answers: see page 176.

63 Lumps in the groin

A	indirect inguinal hernia	G	femoral hernia
B	femoral aneurysm	H	seminoma
C	hydrocele	I	scrotal carcinoma
D	infected lymph node	J	saphena varix
E	direct inguinal hernia	K	calcified lymph node
F	psoas abscess	L	none of the above

For each clinical scenario below, give the most likely cause for the clinical findings. Each option may be used only once.

1   A 45-year-old woman presents with an irreducible lump in the left groin that is positioned below and lateral to the pubic tubercle.

2   A 26-year-old man presents after surgery with a reducible lump in the left groin above and medial to the pubic tubercle. The lump is not controlled after reduction by pressure over the internal inguinal ring.

3   A 40-year-old man presents with a swelling in the right groin that descends into the scrotum. It can be controlled after reduction by pressure over the internal inguinal ring.

4   A 55-year-old woman presents with a soft lump in her left groin. There is an expansile cough impulse and a fluid thrill is felt when percussing lower down the leg.

5   A 60-year-old smoker complains of a throbbing lump in his right groin. Examination reveals an expansile pulsation in the mass.

Answers: see page 177.

64 Pain/lumps in the scrotum

A	epididymal cyst	G	varicocele
B	chronic orchitis	H	direct inguinal hernia
C	ectopic testis	I	acute epididymo-orchitis
D	syphilis	J	testicular aneurysm
E	torsion of testis	K	hydrocele
F	seminoma		

For each clinical scenario below, give the most likely cause for the clinical findings. Each option may be used only once.

1   A 34-year-old man with a history of undescended testes presents with weight loss and a hard painless testicular lump.

2   A 12-year-old boy presents with severe pain in the testis associated with vomiting after jumping on his bicycle.

3   A 25-year-old man presents with a testicular swelling that has increased in size over the last couple of months. The swelling is fluctuant and the underlying testis impalpable.

4   A 45-year-old man presenting with a scrotal swelling is worried that he is growing a third testicle. On examination there is a smooth fluctuant swelling within the scrotum. Both left and right testes are palpable.

5   A 19-year-old man complains of severe pain and swelling of sudden onset in his right scrotum. Testis and epididymis are very tender. He reports that he has had unprotected intercourse recently.

Answers: see page 178.

65 Anorectal conditions

A	fissure *in ano*	G	anal carcinoma
B	perianal warts	H	rectal prolapse
C	proctalgia fugax	I	pruritus ani
D	second-degree haemorrhoids	J	ischiorectal abscess
E	fistula *in ano*	K	third-degree haemorrhoids
F	pilinoidal sinus	L	syphilitic gumma

For each clinical scenario below, give the most likely cause for the clinical findings. Each option may be used only once.

1   A 28-year-old man with Crohn's disease complains of watery discharge from a puckered area 2 cm from the anal canal.

2   A 32-year-old woman who has recently given birth complains of excruciating pain on defecation, which persists for hours afterwards. Examination reveals a defect posterior to the anal canal.

3   A 30-year-old builder complains of a pain and discharge from an area in the midline of the natal cleft about 4 cm above the anus. This problem has been remitting and recurring for 2 years.

4   A 27-year-old pregnant woman presents with constipation and bright-red blood coating her stools. On examination in the lithotomy position, two bluish tender spongy masses are found protruding from the anus. These do not reduce spontaneously and require digital reduction.

5   A 19-year-old woman presents with multiple papilliferous lesions around the anus.

Answers: see page 179.

66 Ulcers

A	basal cell carcinoma	G	ischaemic ulcer
B	Bowen's disease	H	neuropathic ulcer
C	squamous cell carcinoma	I	gumma
D	aphthous ulcer	J	tuberculous ulcer
E	Marjolin's ulcer	K	verruca
F	venous ulcer		

Select from the options above, the type of ulcer that is being described in the questions below. Each option may be used only once.

1   A 62-year-old man presents with a flat sloping-edged ulcer over the left medial malleolus.

2   A tanned 66-year-old man presents with an ulcer on the nose with a rolled edge.

3   A 60-year-old man complains of a bleeding ulcer on the upper region of the left cheek. It has an everted edge and there are some palpable cervical lymph nodes.

4   A 71-year-old man presents with an exquisitely painful punched-out ulcer on the tip of the right big toe. On examination, the surrounding area is cold.

5   A 58-year-old person with diabetes presents with a painless punched-out ulcer on the sole of the right foot. The surrounding area has reduced pain sensation.

Answers: see page 180.

67 Treatment of peripheral vascular disease

A	intravenous heparin	G	Fogarty catheter
B	femoral–popliteal bypass	H	percutaneous transluminal
C	conservative management		angioplasty
D	sympathectomy	I	aortobifemoral bypass
E	femoral–femoral crossover graft	J	above-knee amputation
F	thrombolysis	K	below-knee amputation

For each clinical scenario below, suggest the most appropriate management. Each option may be used only once.

1   A 75-year-old smoker presents with severe rest pain in her right leg. On examination there is advanced gangrene of the right foot with absent pulses distal to the popliteal pulse.

2   A 55-year-old overweight smoker presents with pain in his legs after walking half a mile, which is relieved immediately by rest. Ankle brachial pressure index is 0.8.

3   A 62-year-old man presents with severe bilateral pain in the legs. He is known to suffer from impotence and buttock claudication. Femoral pulses are weak. Arteriography shows stenosis in both common iliac arteries with good distal run-off.

4   A 65-year-old man complains of left calf claudication of 50 m. Angiography reveals a 10-cm stenosis of the superficial femoral artery.

5   A 74-year-old man with atrial fibrillation who suffered a stroke a week ago presents with an ischaemic cold foot. Arteriography reveals that there is an occlusion at the popliteal artery.

Answers: see page 181.

68 Postoperative complications

A	recurrent laryngeal nerve palsy	G	adhesions
B	tracheal obstruction	H	deep vein thrombosis
C	paralytic ileus	I	ischaemic bowel
D	pulmonary embolus	J	pneumonia
E	hypercalcaemia	K	hypokalaemia
F	perforated bowel	L	hypocalcaemia

Choose, from the options above, the postoperative complication that is being described in the questions below. Each option may be used only once.

1   A 40-year-old man presents with a hoarse voice after subtotal thyroidectomy.

2   A 40-year-old woman presents with pain and swelling in her left calf after pelvic surgery.

3   A 62 year old presents with sudden onset shortness of breath 10 days after a hip replacement.

4   A 40-year-old man presents with tetany after a near-total thyroidectomy.

5   A 46-year-old man with a history of bowel surgery presents with abdominal pain and vomiting. On examination there is some tenderness on palpation. Bowel sounds are tinkling. His abdominal radiograph shows dilated loops of small bowel.

Answers: see page 182.

69 Haematuria

A	renal cell carcinoma	G	ureteric calculus
B	Wegener's granulomatosis	H	polycystic kidney disease
C	acute cystitis	I	bladder carcinoma
D	idiopathic haematuria	J	Goodpasture's syndrome
E	benign prostatic hypertrophy	K	carcinoma of prostate
F	post-infectious glomerulonephritis	L	Henoch–Schönlein purpura

For each clinical scenario below, suggest the most likely cause for the haematuria. Each option may be used only once.

1   A 55-year-old smoker presents with painless haematuria and weight loss. Ultrasonography of the kidneys is normal.

2   A 6-year-old boy presents with a 2-week history of non-blanching rash over the buttocks and macroscopic haematuria. He complains of pain in both knees.

3   A 9-year-old boy presents with periorbital oedema and microscopic haematuria plus proteinuria. Anti-streptolysin O titre (ASOT) is positive and serum C3 is reduced. Apart from a sore throat 2 weeks ago, he has no previous medical history of note.

4   A 30-year-old man presents with a colicky loin pain that radiates to the groin area, which is associated with nausea and vomiting.

5   A 75-year-old woman presents with frequency, pain on micturition and haematuria.

Answers: see page 183.

70 Weight loss

A	ulcerative colitis	G	diabetes mellitus
B	diabetes insipidus	H	pancreatic carcinoma
C	tuberculosis	I	thyrotoxicosis
D	renal carcinoma	J	irritable bowel syndrome
E	carcinoma of the stomach	K	anorexia nervosa
F	coeliac disease	L	Crohn's disease

For each clinical scenario below, give the most likely cause for the weight loss. Each option may be used only once.

1. A 26-year-old woman complains of weight loss associated with diarrhoea and palpitations. Her pulse is irregular.

2. A 30-year-old Asian man complains of fever, weight loss, night sweats and persistent cough.

3. A 55-year-old woman presents with abdominal pain, weight loss and fatty stools. She also complains of extremely uncomfortable itchy blisters on her knees and elbows.

4. A 10-year-old boy presents with a history of weight loss and excessive thirst.

5. A 24-year-old woman complains of tiredness and difficulty in concentrating at university. On examination she has marked weight loss and lanugo hair. Blood tests reveal a mild hypokalaemia.

Answers: see page 184.

71 Dysphagia

A bulbar palsy
B pharyngeal pouch
C Plummer–Vinson syndrome
D obstructing foreign body
E seventh nerve palsy
F Sturge–Weber syndrome

G oesophageal achalasia
H retrosternal goitre
I oesophageal carcinoma
J caustic stricture
K diffuse oesophageal spasm
L globus hystericus

For each clinical scenario below, give the most likely cause for the dysphagia. Each option may be used only once.

1 A 35-year-old woman presents with dysphagia for solid and liquids associated with regurgitation and weight loss. Barium swallow shows a dilated tapering oesophagus.

2 A 65-year-old smoker presents with a history of severe oesophagitis and gradually worsening dysphagia.

3 A 28-year-old woman presents with a feeling of a lump in her throat that causes some discomfort on swallowing. Examination and imaging of the pharynx and oesophagus reveal no abnormality.

4 A 40-year-old man complains of intermittent dysphagia associated with chest pain. Barium swallow reveals a corkscrew oesophagus.

5 A 55-year-old man presents coughing when he tries to swallow. On examination he has a flaccid fasciculating tongue.

Answers: see page 185.

72 Lower gastrointestinal bleeding

A   ulcerative colitis
B   Crohn's disease
C   Mallory–Weiss tear
D   haemophilia
E   diverticulosis
F   Meyer–Betz syndrome

G   Peutz–Jeghers syndrome
H   anal fissure
I   infectious diarrhoea
J   colonic carcinoma
K   haemorrhoids
L   intussusception

For each clinical scenario below, give the most likely cause for the bleeding. Each option may be used only once.

1   A 62-year-old man presents with rectal bleeding and a year's history of left iliac fossa pain and change in bowel habit. There is no weight loss.

2   An 8-month-old baby presents with inconsolable crying, colic and bleeding per rectum. A sausage-shaped abdominal mass is palpable.

3   A 35-year-old man returns from holiday with a 2-week history of fever, cramping abdominal pain and bloody diarrhoea.

4   A 60-year-old man complains of tiredness and significant weight loss. He notes episodes of rectal bleeding with blood mixed in with the stool over the last few weeks. There is no diarrhoea.

5   A 21-year-old man presents with a history of constipation and rectal bleeding. On examination there are numerous dark freckles on the palm, lips and oral mucosa.

Answers: see page 186.

73 Haematemesis

A	oesophageal varices	G	Osler–Weber–Rendu syndrome
B	duodenal ulcer	H	gastric carcinoma
C	infectious gastritis	I	gastric ulcer
D	Crohn's disease	J	Barrett's oesophagus
E	Mallory–Weiss tear	K	aortoenteric fistula
F	Peutz–Jeghers syndrome		

For each clinical scenario below, give the most likely cause for the haematemesis. Each option may be used only once.

1   A 50-year-old man who is an alcoholic complains of vomiting blood. On examination he has signs of chronic liver disease.

2   A 55-year-old businessman complains of epigastric pain worse at night which is relieved by eating. He has started vomiting small amounts of blood.

3   A 60-year-old woman with a several year history of heartburn presents with occasional haematemesis. Endoscopy reveals intestinal-type metaplasia at the distal oesophagus.

4   A 40-year-old woman presents with haematemesis after a bout of prolonged vomiting.

5   A 60-year-old woman with pernicious anaemia presents with a 2-month history of dyspepsia, weight loss and haematemesis. Examination reveals an enlarged left supraclavicular node.

Answers: see page 187.

74 Diarrhoea

A   diverticulitis
B   lactose intolerance
C   thyrotoxicosis
D   Crohn's disease
E   inflammatory bowel disease
F   irritable bowel syndrome

G   laxative abuse
H   gastroenteritis
I   pseudomembranous colitis
J   coeliac disease
K   ulcerative colitis
L   cystic fibrosis

For each clinical scenario below, give the most likely cause for the diarrhoea. Each option may be used only once.

1   A 19-year-old backpacker presents with a 2-day history of vomiting and watery diarrhoea.

2   A 75-year-old patient treated with broad-spectrum antibiotics presents a few days later with bloody diarrhoea.

3   An anxious 31-year-old woman complains of a history of chronic diarrhoea alternating with constipation. She often feels bloated. Investigations are normal.

4   A 17-year-old man presents with symptoms of chronic diarrhoea and smelly stools. He has a history of recurrent chest infections as a child.

5   A 35-year-old woman with diabetes presents with weight loss, diarrhoea and angular stomatitis. Blood tests reveal presence of anti-gliadin antibodies.

Answers: see page 188.

75 Constipation

A	hypothyroidism	G	hyperkalaemia
B	hypokalaemia	H	ferrous sulphate
C	irritable bowel syndrome	I	hypercalcaemia
D	caecal carcinoma	J	colorectal carcinoma
E	Chagas' disease	K	diverticular disease
F	folate supplements		

For each clinical scenario below, give the most likely cause for the constipation.
Each option may be used only once.

1   An 80-year-old woman presents with thirst, tiredness, depression, bone pain and
     constipation.

2   A 65-year-old man presents with a 3-month history of weight loss, altered
     bowel habit and bleeding per rectum.

3   A 42-year-old woman complains of weight gain, constipation, cold intolerance
     and depression.

4   A 65-year-old woman presents with constipation and colicky left-sided
     abdominal pain relieved by defecation.

5   A 21-year-old woman presenting with weakness and lethargy has been success-
     fully treated for anaemia. She now complains of constipation and black stools.

Answers: see page 189.

76 Abnormal abdominal radiographs

A	Crohn's disease	G	sigmoid volvulus
B	diverticulosis	H	intussusception
C	chronic pancreatitis	I	ulcerative colitis
D	acute pancreatitis	J	pyloric stenosis
E	gluten-sensitive enteropathy	K	small bowel obstruction
F	acute appendicitis	L	perforated ulcer

For each clinical scenario below, give the most likely cause for the clinical findings. Each option may be used only once.

1   A 55 year old with a history of epigastric discomfort of several months presents acutely unwell in A&E. His radiograph shows free gas under the diaphragm.

2   Abdominal film of an elderly constipated woman shows an 'inverted U' loop of bowel.

3   A 31-year-old man presents with fever and bloody diarrhoea. He is tachycardic and has a Hb of 10.0 g/dl. Abdominal film shows loss of haustral pattern and a colonic dilatation of 8 cm.

4   A 26-year-old student presents with bloody diarrhoea, abdominal pain and weight loss. Barium enema reveals 'cobble-stoning' and colonic strictures.

5   A 45-year-old man presents with severe epigastric pain and vomiting. Abdominal film shows absent psoas shadow and 'sentinel loop' of proximal jejunum.

Answers: see page 190.

77 Treatment of gastrointestinal conditions

A	high-dose lansoprazole	G	intravenous hydrocortisone
B	ibuprofen four times daily	H	mebeverine
C	clarithromycin, amoxicillin, lansoprazole	I	morphine
		J	endoscopy
D	intravenous prednisolone	K	intravenous fluids only
E	laparotomy	L	clarithromycin, amoxicillin
F	low-dose omeprazole		

For each clinical scenario below, suggest the most appropriate management. Each option may be used only once.

1   A 50-year-old man presenting with a perforated gastric ulcer.

2   A 55-year-old woman with severe oesophagitis confirmed on endoscopy.

3   A 60-year-old man with cirrhosis presenting with haematemesis.

4   A 30-year-old man with ulcerative colitis presents to A&E with fever, tachycardia and abdominal distension.

5   A 24-year-old woman with suspected irritable bowel syndrome complains of colicky pain and bloating.

Answers: see page 191.

ANSWERS

54 Abdominal pain

Answers: B K F E J

> A 45-year-old man with a history of gallstones presents in A&E with severe epigastric pain radiating to the back and vomiting.

B   Severe epigastric pain radiating to the back is the classic description of acute pancreatitis, and gallstones and alcohol are its two most common causes. Serum amylase is usually significantly raised but this is not specific because amylase can be raised with other conditions that present with an acute abdomen, such as cholecystitis and perforated viscus.

> A 28-year-old man presents with sharp left loin and left upper quadrant pain radiating to the groin. He is not jaundiced.

K   Renal colic is severe and often associated with nausea and vomiting. It is very important to provide adequate analgesia and morphine may be required.

> A 44-year-old woman presents with continuous right upper quadrant pain, vomiting and fever. Murphy's sign is positive.

F   Murphy's sign is an indicator of acute cholecystitis. The hand is placed over the right upper quadrant and the patient is asked to breathe in. The pain resulting from the inflamed gallbladder moving downwards and striking the hand is severe and arrests the inspiratory effort.

> A 26-year-old man with a previous history of abdominal surgery presents with colicky central abdominal pain, rapidly followed by production of copious bile-stained vomitus.

E   There is usually early onset of vomiting and late development of distension in small bowel obstruction. An abdominal radiograph may show distended loops proximal to the obstruction and lack of gas in the large bowel. In large bowel obstruction vomiting only occurs later and is faeculent (mixed with faeces).

> A 50-year-old man presents with epigastric pain worse at night and relieved by eating or drinking milk.

J   Classically the pain of duodenal ulceration is described as being relieved by eating, whereas the pain of gastric ulceration is described as worsening on eating. In practice it is difficult to identify the site of ulceration based on such information.

Helicobacter pylori infection and chronic non-steroidal anti-inflammatory drug (NSAID) use are important risk factors for duodenal ulceration. Nearly all duodenal ulcers are *Helicobacter pylori* positive.

55 Abdominal pain

Answers: B E K H A

A 21-year-old student presents with a cramping diffuse abdominal pain associated with alternating constipation and diarrhoea. Investigations are normal.

B   Irritable bowel syndrome is associated with a stressful lifestyle. Younger women (under 40) are more frequently affected. The patient may report pain relief after defecating/passing flatus.

A 55-year-old smoker presents with severe epigastric pain. The chest radiograph reveals air under the diaphragm.

E   Air under the diaphragm can be seen with any perforated viscus.

A 9-year-old girl presents with fever, nausea and right iliac fossa pain. She says that the pain 'was around my belly-button before'.

K   This is a classic presentation of appendicitis, with a central colicky abdominal pain that shifts to the right iliac fossa once the peritoneum becomes inflamed. Rebound tenderness can be elicited with appendicitis. As the appendix may lie in various positions (e.g. retrocaecal, paracaecal, retrocolic, pelvic), pain may sometimes be elicited by rectal/vaginal examination. Treatment involves prompt appendicectomy.

A 35-year-old man presents with weight loss, diarrhoea and abdominal pain. On examination, he has aphthous ulcers in the mouth and a mass is palpable in the right iliac fossa. Blood tests reveal low serum vitamin B_{12} and folate.

H   Crohn's disease is a chronic transmural inflammatory gastrointestinal disease that can result in skip lesions anywhere from the mouth (aphthous ulceration) to the anus (e.g. fissuring/fistulae), but favours the terminal ileum/proximal colon. Small bowel disease can lead to malabsorption, e.g. iron, vitamin B_{12} and folate.

A 45-year-old woman on treatment for TB presents with abdominal pain and malaise. On examination she is jaundiced.

A   Pyrazinamide, isoniazid and rifampicin are all recognized causes of drug-induced hepatitis. Remember that rifampicin is commonly associated with a transient elevation in hepatic transaminases, but this does not indicate the development of full-blown hepatitis and so withdrawal of treatment is not necessarily indicated.

56 Abdominal masses

Answers: K C I E F

> A 65-year-old man collapses in the street. On examination he has an umbilical mass that is expansile and pulsatile.

K The presence of an expansile and pulsatile mass implies the presence of an aneurysm. A true aneurysm is lined by all three layers of the arterial wall, whereas a false aneurysm (caused by trauma, infection, etc.) is lined only by connective tissue. The UK Small Aneurysm Trial suggested that elective surgical repair of aneurysm is indicated with an aneurysm diameter greater than 5.5 cm (Mortality results from randomised controlled trial of early elective surgery or ultrasonographic surveillance for small abdominal aortic aneurysms. *Lancet* 1998; 352: 1649–55). Early elective surgery may prevent rupture although the mortality rate is 5–6 per cent. Operative options include replacement with a prosthetic graft or endovascular stent graft repair. Ultrasonographic surveillance for small abdominal aortic aneurysms is safe and early surgery provides a long-term survival advantage.

The mortality rate from aneurysm rupture without surgery is 100 per cent and even if the patient reaches the hospital surgical unit alive, the overall mortality rate is very high (80–95 per cent).

> A 75-year-old man with a 3-month history of dyspepsia presents with weight loss and abdominal distension. On examination a 3.5 cm, hard, irregular, tender epigastric mass can be felt which moves on respiration. Percussion of the distended abdomen reveals shifting dullness. The left supraclavicular node is palpable.

C Gastric carcinoma should always be considered in a patient complaining of dyspepsia for over a month in someone this age. The presence of Virchow's node (left supraclavicular node) and ascites implies disseminated disease and thus carries a poor prognosis. This finding is sometimes referred to as a positive Troisier's sign.

> A 70-year-old woman presents with a mass in the right iliac fossa and severe microcytic anaemia. On examination the mass is firm, irregular and 4 cm in diameter. The lower edge is palpable.

I The predominant symptoms/signs of carcinoma vary depending on the site of colon affected. Right-sided lesions in the caecum/ascending colon are associated with weight loss and anaemia, whereas symptoms of change in bowel habit and bleeding per rectum are more common in the sigmoid colon/rectum. The possibility of a caecal carcinoma must always be considered in a patient over 40 years of age presenting with acute appendicitis.

A 35-year-old woman is worried about an abdominal mass that has grown over the last 6 months and a similar length history of very heavy menstrual bleeding with no intermenstrual bleeding. On examination a knobbly mass can be felt in the middle lower quadrant that is dull to percussion. The lower edge is not palpable. She is otherwise well.

E Fibroids are the commonly used name for fibromyomas, which are benign tumours of uterine smooth muscle. The incidence of fibroids increases with age.

Patients typically present with symptoms of increased menstrual blood loss in middle-aged women. Other common presentations include infertility and symptoms caused by pressure on other structures, e.g. urinary frequency, constipation. Fibroids vary considerably in size and may grow such that they occupy a large part of the abdomen and compress other structures. A patient may also present with an acute abdomen after thrombosis of a fibroid's blood supply (red degeneration).

Management depends on several factors, including the size of the fibroids, symptoms, patient's circumstances, etc. Surgical interventions include myomectomy, uterine artery embolism and hysterectomy. Fibroids are oestrogen dependent and gonadotrophin analogues are sometimes given to shrink fibroids before surgery.

A 70 year old with alcohol problems presents with a tender upper abdominal mass. CT shows a thick-walled, rounded, fluid-filled mass adjacent to the pancreas.

F Pancreatic pseudocysts are usually located in the lesser sac adjacent to the pancreas. They occur as a result of ductal leakage after inflammation of the pancreas (acute or chronic). Chronic pancreatitis is the most common cause of pancreatic pseudocyst. These patients may present nonspecifically with abdominal discomfort, nausea, early satiety, etc.

Complications of pancreatic pseudocyst include infection (most common), obstruction (of common bile duct leading to jaundice) and perforation. Very rarely the pseudocyst can enlarge such that it erodes nearby vessels, causing pseudoaneurysm formation that can be fatal. Fortunately, most pseudocysts resolve spontaneously.

CT is the investigation of choice and typically shows a round/ovoid fluid-filled cavity encapsulated by a fibrous wall. A pseudocyst does not have a true epithelial lining. Pancreatic pseudocysts can be treated by drainage if it is felt that there is a high risk of complication.

57 Liver diseases

Answers: A K E H D

A 69-year-old retired bricklayer presents with weight loss, fever and right upper quadrant pain. On examination, a hard, irregular liver can be felt on palpation. Serum AFP is grossly elevated.

A   Liver metastases and conditions associated with a macronodular cirrhosis
       may give rise to a hard irregular liver. The significantly raised
       α-fetoprotein (AFP) is suggestive of hepatocellular carcinoma. Hepatitis
       and chronic cardiac failure are usually associated with a smooth rather
       than an irregular hepatomegaly.

       **A 45-year-old man presents with arthralgia, tiredness and develop-
       ment of diabetes. On examination his skin is pigmented and blood
       tests show increased serum ferritin.**

K   Haemochromatosis is an autosomal recessively inherited disorder of iron
       metabolism that most commonly presents in middle-aged men. The
       presentation can be very non-specific in the early stages, e.g. lethargy,
       joint pain. Later the classic features of chronic liver disease and 'bronze
       diabetes' (hence pigmentation) may become apparent. Haemochromatosis
       can also cause a dilated cardiomyopathy, resulting in heart failure.
       Blood tests show a raised serum iron and ferritin with decreased total
       iron-binding capacity.
       Radiographs of the painful joints may show signs of chondrocalcinosis.
       Venesection plays an important role in long-term management to
       maintain the haematocrit and ferritin within normal ranges.

       **A 60-year-old publican presents with signs of spider naevi, gynaeco-
       mastia and testicular atrophy. His hands show clubbing and leukonychia.**

E   Other signs of chronic liver disease include Dupuytren's contracture,
       palmar erythema and parotid enlargement.

       **A 20-year-old man with a history of liver problems in the past
       presents with tremor and dysarthria with developing dyskinesias.
       Slit-lamp examination reveals a greenish-brown ring at the
       corneoscleral junction.**

H   Wilson's disease is an autosomal recessive condition characterized by
       toxic accumulation of copper in the liver and brain. The characteristic
       eye sign described in the question is a Kaiser–Fleischer ring, which is
       best observed under slit-lamp examination and is virtually
       pathognomonic of Wilson's disease. It is a greenish-brown ring that
       can be seen at the corneoscleral junction. It is caused by copper
       deposition in Descemet's membrane.
       Neurological problems may manifest as dementia, tremor, dyskinesias, etc.
       Management of Wilson's disease involves long-term treatment with a
       copper-chelating agent such as penicillamine.

       **A 50-year-old man presents with signs of chronic liver disease with a
       history of early onset pulmonary emphysema. He is a non-smoker
       and is teetotal. His father had a similar history.**

D α_1-Antitrypsin deficiency is an autosomally dominant inherited condi-
       tion that characteristically affects the lungs and the liver. Pulmonary

emphysema and its complications are the major cause of mortality in these individuals.

The most common pattern of emphysema that is seen in hospitals is a centrilobular/centriacinar emphysema which is smoking related. The damage is predominantly in the respiratory bronchioles with relative preservation of the alveoli.

However, α_1-antitrypsin deficiency is associated with a much rarer panacinar emphysema that involves the destruction of whole alveoli and predominantly affects the lung bases. As smoking promotes the inactivation of α_1-antitrypsin, it results in the patient developing emphysema earlier.

58 Causes of splenomegaly

Answers: L E H A J

> A 75-year-old woman with long-standing rheumatoid arthritis is seen to have splenomegaly on abdominal examination. Her full blood count shows anaemia and a low white cell count.

L   Felty's syndrome is a condition characterized by splenomegaly and neutropenia in a patient with rheumatoid arthritis (RA). It is strongly associated with HLA-DR4 genotype and patients are usually very strongly rheumatoid factor positive. Management involves treating the underlying RA. If patients do not improve with medical therapy and have recurrent infections, splenectomy may be indicated.

> A 35-year-old man presents with an insidious onset of hepatosplenomegaly with marked pigmentation on the forehead and hands. He is anaemic and has a history of pathological fractures.

E   Gaucher's disease is a lysosomal storage disease that results from glucocerebrosidase deficiency and a consequent accumulation of glucosylceramide in the lysosomes of the reticuloendothelial system. There is a notably high incidence in Ashkenazi Jews.

The history in this question is suggestive of type I disease (types II and III are associated with significant neurological involvement), which usually involves a presentation with anaemia, hepatosplenomegaly and symptoms relating to bone involvement. Patients are also found to have increased pigmentation, particularly on the forehead and hands. Bone involvement gives rise to pathological fractures. Radiographs may reveal some classic bone-modelling deformities, e.g. 'Erlenmeyer's flask' in which the end of a long bone is expanded and the shaft has a straightened/convex margin. Osteonecrosis and painful lytic lesions are also common.

Bone marrow biopsy is used for diagnosis to identify the pathognomonic Gaucher cells. Treatment involves enzyme replacement therapy.

A 23-year-old man presents with a week's history of fever and sore throat. He developed a macular rash after being prescribed ampicillin by his GP. On examination he has enlarged posterior cervical nodes, palatal petechiae and splenomegaly.

H   Infectious mononucleosis is more commonly known as glandular fever and results from primary infection with Epstein–Barr virus (EBV). The appearance of a faint morbilliform eruption or maculopapular rash after the patient is treated with ampicillin is a characteristic sign of EBV infection. There is a T-cell proliferation, with the presence of large atypical cells that can be observed on the blood film. There is no antiviral therapy and the patient is simply advised to rest for uncomplicated infection. Complications are rare but include thrombocytopenia, aseptic meningitis and Guillain–Barré syndrome.

A 21-year-old female backpacker returning from India presents with flu-like symptoms followed by a periodic fever. She is anaemic, jaundiced and has moderate splenomegaly.

A   The fever of malaria is classically periodic, e.g. peaking every third day. This is caused by rupture of infected erythrocytes releasing matured merozoites and pyrogens. This classic paroxysm may not necessarily be present in early infection.
Thick and thin blood smears are required for diagnosis. Resistance to the traditional quinine-based drugs is now widespread and newer drugs are in development.

A 28-year-old woman presents with abdominal pain, vomiting and jaundice. On examination she has tender hepatomegaly and ascites. She has a history of recurrent miscarriages.

J   Budd–Chiari syndrome is a condition characterized by obstruction to hepatic venous outflow. It usually occurs in a patient with a hypercoagulative state (e.g. antiphospholipid syndrome, use of oral contraceptive pill, malignancy) but can also occur as a result of physical obstruction, e.g. tumour. The venous congestion can lead to enlargement of the spleen as well as the liver. The history of recurrent miscarriages suggests that there may be an underlying disorder, e.g. antiphospholipid syndrome, and this should be investigated thoroughly.

59 Jaundice

Answers: C A J L M

A 24 year old presents with nausea, malaise and jaundice. He returned 3 weeks ago from a holiday abroad. On examination he has a moderate hepatosplenomegaly and tender cervical lymphadenopathy. He has dark urine and pale stools.

C   Hepatitis A is an RNA virus that is spread by the faecal–oral route. It is particularly associated with travellers. Treatment is supportive because the condition is usually self-limiting.

A 35-year-old woman presents with fever, malaise and jaundice. On examination she has moderate hepatomegaly. She is anti-smooth muscle antibody and antinuclear antibody positive.

A   Chronic autoimmune hepatitis occurs most frequently in women and has associations with many other autoimmune diseases. Type I disease is associated with the presence of antinuclear and/or anti-smooth muscle antibodies.
        Immunosuppressive therapy, e.g. corticosteroids, azathioprin, can induce remission in most cases. The patient may eventually require liver transplantation (recurrence after transplantation is still possible).

A 25-year-old man presents with recurrent episodes of asymptomatic jaundice.

J   Patients with Gilbert's syndrome may describe a family history of asymptomatic jaundice. This condition involves an unconjugated hyper-bilirubinaemia where a rise in bilirubin is seen particularly on fasting, dehydration, illness, etc. It is thought to result from underactivity of UDP-glucuronyl transferase activity, an enzyme involved in the conjugation of bilirubin. It is important to educate patients that there is no underlying liver disease and that Gilbert's syndrome is essentially a benign condition.

A 4-year-old patient presents with anaemia and mild jaundice. Hb 7 g/dl, reticulocytes 14 per cent. Electrophoresis result pending.

L   Markers of haemolytic anaemia on a peripheral blood film include reticulocytosis (caused by increased erythrocyte production), elevated serum unconjugated bilirubin, reduced plasma haptoglobin and increased urinary urobilinogen. Remember that urinary urobilinogen is absent in cholestatic jaundice.

A 45-year-old man with ulcerative colitis presents with jaundice, pruritus and abdominal pain. ALP is raised and anti-mitochondrial antibodies negative.

M   Anti-mitochondrial antibodies are associated with primary biliary cirrhosis not primary sclerosing cholangitis. There is an association of primary sclerosing cholangitis with HLA-B8 and -DR3. The fibrosis and stricturing of the biliary tree give rise to a beaded appearance on endoscopic retrograde cholangiopancreatography (ERCP).

60 Breast conditions

Answers: F M H A K

A 75-year-old woman presents to her GP with a breast lump in the upper outer quadrant. On examination the lump is hard and irregular. There is axillary lymphadenopathy.

F A hard irregular lump is a cause for concern and warrants further investigation.

A 53-year-old woman presents with nipple retraction and a greeny-yellow discharge. Her ductogram shows dilated breast ducts.

M Duct ectasia is a condition that usually occurs peri-/postmenopausally. It has been suggested that there is hypertrophy of the ductal epithelium, which subsequently breaks down and causes obstruction (and hence stagnation of secretions). There is periductal inflammation that can lead to fibrosis and nipple retraction. It is important to rule out carcinoma especially as a mass or blood-stained discharge can also be seen in duct ectasia. A ductogram characteristically shows the presence of enlarged, dilated breast ducts.

A 21-year-old woman presents with a smooth, non-tender, highly mobile mass on the upper outer quadrant of the right breast. Fine needle aspiration does not reveal malignant features.

H Fibroadenomas are characteristically highly mobile and have the consistency of firm rubber. This has given rise to the description of a fibroadenoma as a 'breast mouse'. A fibroadenoma has the appearance of a well-defined rounded lesion on mammogram. Fibroadenomas should be excised not only to confirm the diagnosis (particularly as an early carcinoma in older women may mimic a fibroadenoma) but also because they enlarge over time.

A 70-year-old woman presents with a worsening eczema-like rash overlying the areola and nipple. The rash does not itch. On examination a palpable mass can be felt under the rash.

A This condition is caused by an intraductal carcinoma, which spreads up to the skin of the nipple causing eczematous changes. There is gradual erosion and ulceration of the nipple. Fortunately, as the carcinoma is superficial and presentation is early (because of the eczematous changes), the prognosis is good.

A 26-year-old woman presents a fortnight post partum with a painful, enlarged left breast. On examination she is pyrexial and her breast is tender and inflamed. There are no palpable masses.

K Inflammation of the breast post partum can be caused by obstruction of the ducts, resulting in extravasation of milk into perilobular tissue.

This usually occurs a few days post partum and is self-limiting. Presentation a few weeks after delivery, with a more persistent pyrexia and the presence of purulent discharge, implies the presence of infective mastitis. It is important to stop direct breast-feeding of the child and send a sample of the breast milk for microscopy, culture and sensitivity. As *Staphylococcus aureus* is by far the most common infective agent, flucloxacillin treatment can be started in the meantime. The major complication of mastitis is the development of an abscess, which is managed surgically by incision and drainage.

61 Presentation with a lump

Answers: I E C H L

A 22-year-old man presents with a lump on the scalp. Examination reveals a smooth, spherical, tense lump. A small punctum can be seen on the surface.

I Sebaceous cysts can occur anywhere where there are sebaceous glands. There are no sebaceous glands on the palms of the hand and the soles of the feet. The scalp is a commonly affected area. The punctum visible on the surface of the lump is virtually diagnostic of sebaceous cyst.

A 33-year-old man presents with a swelling on the upper arm that has been growing slowly for a number of years. Examination reveals a soft, compressible, non-tender, lobulated mass.

E This is a typical history of lipoma with slow growth over a number of years. The lobulation is diagnostically important.

A 28-year-old man presents with a painless swelling on the dorsum of the right hand. Examination reveals a smooth, spherical, tense, 1.5 cm swelling. The overlying skin can be drawn over it.

C A ganglion is a cystic degeneration of fibrous tissue and is usually found around joints, especially the dorsal surface of the wrist joint. Treatment is by excision under general anaesthetic.

A 29-year-old man presents with two mobile fusiform-shaped lumps on the forearm. Each swelling feels like firm rubber and causes tingling in the hand on pressure.

H Neurofibromas are often multiple and can appear at any age, but usually present in adult life. The forearm is frequently affected. The presence of multiple neurofibromas may indicate the presence of neurofibromatosis (look out for café-au-lait spots, Lisch nodules in the eye, acoustic neuroma, etc.). These patients need to be followed up because there is a risk of sarcomatous change.

A 65-year-old woman presents with a rapidly growing lump just below the eye. Examination reveals a 2 cm smooth, round, skin-coloured lump with a black central core. The lump is freely mobile over subcutaneous tissues.

L Keratoacanthoma (also known as molluscum sebaceum) is caused by benign overgrowth of a sebaceous gland and is often mistaken for squamous cell carcinoma. Squamous cell carcinoma does not have the central necrotic core. A keratoacanthoma should always be mobile over subcutaneous tissues.

62 Lumps in the neck

Answers: B E L A G

A 28-year-old man presents with halitosis and regurgitation of food. He has a lump in the posterior triangle.

B A pharyngeal pouch is a pulsion diverticulum of pharyngeal mucosa between the thyropharyngeal and cricopharyngeal muscles. There is a higher incidence of pharyngeal pouch in men. On examination the lump can be compressed and sometimes emptied. The swelling is positioned behind the sternocleidomastoid muscle. Diagnosis can be made by barium swallow and treatment involves excision of the pouch (a cricopharyngeal myotomy is also carried out to prevent recurrence).

A 20-year-old woman presents with a small painless midline swelling that has increased in size. The swelling moves upwards on protruding the tongue.

E The swelling is closely associated with the hyoid bone and thus moves upwards on tongue protrusion. The cyst can appear anywhere between the base of the tongue and the isthmus of the thyroid gland. In practice thyroglossal cysts are usually found either between isthmus and hyoid bone or just above the hyoid bone.

An 8-year-old girl presents with a painful lump just below the angle of the jaw. She has a sore throat and is pyrexial.

L The tonsils drain to the upper deep cervical lymph nodes and thus infection can give rise to tenderness in this area. A general examination is important to identify any lymphadenopathy in other regions.

A 22-year-old man presents with a lump behind the anterior border of sternocleidomastoid on the upper left side of the neck. He has had the lump for a number of years but it has recently become painful.

A Branchial cysts are usually painless unless there is infection involved. The back of the cyst is deep to the sternocleidomastoid and it is not very mobile because it is attached to/closely associated with surrounding structures.

A parent brings a 4-year-old boy to clinic with a large swelling at the base of the posterior triangle. The swelling is soft and fluctuant and transilluminates brilliantly.

G A cystic hygroma is a congenital collection of lymphatic sacs. The distinctive sign is the brilliant transilluminance.

63 Lumps in the groin

Answers: G E A J B

A 45-year-old woman presents with an irreducible lump in the left groin that is positioned below and lateral to the pubic tubercle.

G Femoral hernias are palpable below and lateral to the pubic tubercle, whereas inguinal hernias can be felt above and medial to this landmark. Femoral hernias are often irreducible and likely to strangulate.

A 26-year-old man presents after surgery with a reducible lump in the left groin above and medial to the pubic tubercle. The lump is not controlled after reduction by pressure over the internal inguinal ring.

E Direct hernias push *directly* through the posterior wall of the inguinal canal and thus pressure over the internal ring after reduction will not stop it popping back through the wall. They often reduce easily and rarely strangulate.

A 40-year-old man presents with a swelling in the right groin that descends into the scrotum. It can be controlled after reduction by pressure over the internal inguinal ring.

A Indirect inguinal hernias pass through the internal inguinal ring and therefore can be controlled by pressure over the internal inguinal ring after the hernia has been reduced. Generally speaking, direct inguinal hernias are not felt in the scrotum.

A 55-year-old woman presents with a soft lump in her left groin. There is an expansile cough impulse and a fluid thrill is felt when percussing lower down the leg.

J This is a compressible dilatation at the top of the saphenous vein.

A 60-year-old smoker complains of a throbbing lump in his right groin. Examination reveals an expansile pulsation in the mass.

B Direct pressure of a femoral aneurysm on the femoral vein can lead to venous obstruction and thrombosis. Common femoral artery aneurysms are usually caused by atherosclerotic disease. However, a false aneurysm can be caused via trauma, e.g. a stab wound to the artery. For example, if a patient is stabbed in the femoral artery, a haematoma develops outside the artery and eventually a thrombus occludes the hole in the arterial wall.

The pressure in the artery may force this plug outwards into the haematoma to form a small cavity inside it. This gives rise to the appearance of an expansile and pulsatile mass and is indistinguishable on clinical examination (if history of trauma is not known).

64 Pain/lumps in the scrotum

Answers: F E K A I

> A 34-year-old man with a history of undescended testes presents with weight loss and a hard painless testicular lump.

F   Seminoma usually presents between the age of 30 and 40 years whereas teratoma commonly presents earlier (20–30 years). Undescended testes are an important risk factor for testicular tumours.

> A 12-year-old boy presents with severe pain in the testis associated with vomiting after jumping on his bicycle.

E   There is a congenital anatomical abnormality that allows torsion of the whole testicle. A normal testicle is fixed within the tunica vaginalis and cannot twist. The pain of torsion is severe and often associated with nausea and vomiting. Testicular torsion is a urological emergency and prompt surgical intervention is indicated to ensure salvage of the affected testis. Acute epididymo-orchitis can give a similar presentation, but it is always best to explore surgically to rule out torsion if there is any doubt.
It is important to remember that torsion of the testis can occur spontaneously without any history of trauma.

> A 25-year-old man presents with a testicular swelling that has increased in size over the last couple of months. The swelling is fluctuant and the underlying testis impalpable.

K   As the fluid of the hydrocele surrounds the body of the testis, the underlying testis is impalpable. Primary hydrocele is idiopathic. Secondary hydrocele occurs secondary to trauma, tumour and infection.

> A 45-year-old man presenting with a scrotal swelling is worried that he is growing a third testicle. On examination there is a smooth fluctuant swelling within the scrotum. Both left and right testes are palpable.

A   An epididymal cyst is separate from the testis and therefore the testis is palpable.

> A 19-year-old man complains of severe pain and swelling of sudden onset in his right scrotum. Testis and epididymis are very tender. He reports that he has had unprotected intercourse recently.

I There may be signs of urinary tract infection, i.e. frequency and dysuria. *Chlamydia* sp. and other sources of sexually transmitted infection are more common in younger men whereas bacteria such as *Escherichia coli* are more common in older men.

65 Anorectal conditions

Answers: E A F K B

  A 28-year-old man with Crohn's disease complains of watery discharge from a puckered area 2 cm from the anal canal.

E Fistulae are a well-recognized complication of Crohn's disease. A full rectal examination is important to detect other causes of fistula *in ano*, e.g. rectal carcinoma.

  A 32-year-old woman who has recently given birth complains of excruciating pain on defecation, which persists for hours afterwards. Examination reveals a defect posterior to the anal canal.

A This condition is very painful and frequently means that a rectal examination is not possible. The patient is often constipated because defecation is so painful. This results in a vicious cycle as the stools become harder, resulting in defecation becoming more difficult and painful.

  A 30-year-old builder complains of a pain and discharge from an area in the midline of the natal cleft about 4 cm above the anus. This problem has been remitting and recurring for 2 years.

F Pilinoidal sinuses always occur in the midline of the natal cleft. They are more common in men than in women.

  A 27-year-old pregnant woman presents with constipation and bright-red blood coating her stools. On examination in the lithotomy position, two bluish tender spongy masses are found protruding from the anus. These do not reduce spontaneously and require digital reduction.

K Spongy vascular tissue surrounds and helps close the anal canal. However, if these cushions enlarge they can prolapse and bleed to form haemorrhoids/piles.
First-degree haemorrhoids remain in the rectum.
Second-degree haemorrhoids prolapse through the rectum on defecation but spontaneously reduce.
Third-degree haemorrhoids can be reduced only with digital reduction.
Fourth-degree haemorrhoids remain prolapsed.
Constipation resulting in prolonged straining is a common cause and so a high-fibre diet may be a useful preventive measure.

A 19-year-old woman presents with multiple papilliferous lesions around the anus.

B   Human papilloma virus (HPV) infection is responsible for anogenital warts and is particularly associated with unprotected sexual contact. Also, look out for appearance of such lesions in immunocompromised individuals. HPV-related warts are referred to as condylomata acuminata. Condyloma lata are broad-based, flat-topped and necrotic papules that occur with secondary syphilis. On examination of perianal warts it is important to differentiate the two lesions. If there is any doubt, a biopsy should be performed.

66 Ulcers

Answers: F A C G H

A 62-year-old man presents with a flat sloping-edged ulcer over the left medial malleolus.

F   Venous ulcers are usually found around the lower third of the leg. It is important to remember that in a long-standing venous ulcer there may be malignant change to form a squamous cell carcinoma. This is known as a Marjolin's ulcer.

A tanned 66-year-old man presents with an ulcer on the nose with a rolled edge.

A   Basal cell carcinoma (also known as a rodent ulcer) is a locally invasive carcinoma that is more common on areas of sun-exposed skin. The carcinoma starts as a slow-growing nodule that may be itchy or sometimes bleeds. There is necrosis of the centre, leaving a rolled edge. Basal cell carcinoma does not metastasize and surrounding lymph nodes should not be enlarged.

A 60-year-old man complains of a bleeding ulcer on the upper region of the left cheek. It has an everted edge and there are some palpable cervical lymph nodes.

C   Bleeding is more common in squamous cell carcinoma than in basal cell carcinoma and, unlike the latter, there may be enlarged lymph nodes. Squamous cell carcinoma has a characteristic everted edge.

A 71-year-old man presents with an exquisitely painful punched-out ulcer on the tip of the right big toe. On examination, the surrounding area is cold.

G   Ischaemic ulcers can be excruciatingly painful, to the extent that changing the overlying dressing can lead to pain that lasts for several hours afterwards. Ischaemic ulcers are characteristically deeper than venous ulcers and can penetrate down to the bone. The surrounding area is cold as a result of ischaemia.

A 58-year-old person with diabetes presents with a painless punched-out ulcer on the sole of the right foot. The surrounding area has reduced pain sensation.

H   Neuropathic ulcers occur as a result of impaired sensation caused by neurological deficit of whatever cause. Diabetes mellitus is the most common cause of neuropathic ulcers. They are characteristically painless.

67 Treatment of peripheral vascular disease

Answers: K C I B G

A 75-year-old smoker presents with severe rest pain in her right leg. On examination there is advanced gangrene of the right foot with absent pulses distal to the popliteal pulse.

K   It is especially important to counsel the patient adequately for such a measure. A below-knee amputation is indicated here because there is considerable risk of systemic infection and advancement of the gangrene. The signs of critical limb ischaemia are sometimes summarized as the six 'P's: pain, paraesthesia, pallor, pulselessness, paralysis and perishing with cold.

A 55-year-old overweight smoker presents with pain in his legs after walking half a mile, which is relieved immediately by rest. Ankle brachial pressure index is 0.8.

C   This patient has a relatively large claudication distance (distance travelled before he gets pain) which implies that he does not require invasive treatment.
Ankle brachial pressure index of above 0.9 is normal. Patients with claudication but no rest pain usually have a value that is between 0.6 and 0.9. A value below 0.6 is associated with rest pain and critical ischaemia. Cessation of smoking, more exercise and weight reduction are useful initial measures for the patient in this scenario.
Medical intervention includes the treatment of diabetes, hypertension and hyperlipidaemia.
Daily low-dose aspirin is indicated.

A 62-year-old man presents with severe bilateral pain in the legs. He is known to suffer from impotence and buttock claudication. Femoral pulses are weak. Arteriography shows stenosis in both common iliac arteries with good distal run-off.

I   The distal aorta bifurcates into the two common iliac arteries (the median sacral branch is also given off). The common iliac artery divides to form the external and internal iliac arteries. The external iliac artery passes under the inguinal ligament to become the femoral artery. An aorto-bifemoral bypass will thus provide better circulation distal to the occlusions/narrowing.

A 65-year-old man complains of left calf claudication of 50 m. Angiography reveals a 10-cm stenosis of the superficial femoral artery.

B   The superficial femoral artery becomes the popliteal artery in the popliteal fossa. A femoral–popliteal bypass is the treatment of choice for this scenario where there is significant occlusive disease of the superficial femoral artery.

A 74-year-old man with atrial fibrillation who suffered a stroke a week ago presents with an ischaemic cold foot. Arteriography reveals that there is an occlusion at the popliteal artery.

G   With acute ischaemia secondary to embolism, surgical embolectomy with a Fogarty catheter is indicated. Intra-arterial local thrombolysis involves the use of thrombolytics such as streptokinase/t-PA (tissue plasminogen activator). Thrombolysis would be contraindicated in this trauma scenario because of the patient's recent history of stroke.

68 Postoperative complications

Answers: A H D L G

A 40-year-old man presents with a hoarse voice after subtotal thyroidectomy.

A   The recurrent laryngeal nerve is prone to being stretched or cut during thyroid surgery as a result especially of its close relation to the inferior thyroid artery. A patient with a recurrent laryngeal palsy may complain of dyspnoea on exertion if the cord is fixed in an adducted position.

A 40-year-old woman presents with pain and swelling in her left calf after pelvic surgery.

H   Early mobilization where possible and the use of compressive stockings are important measures in reducing the risk of deep vein thrombosis (DVT).

A 62 year old presents with sudden onset shortness of breath 10 days after a hip replacement.

D   Pelvic surgery and orthopaedic surgery are major risk factors for thromboembolic events such as pulmonary embolism (PE) and DVT.

A 40-year-old man presents with tetany after a near-total thyroidectomy.

L   Hypocalcaemia resulting from a hypoparathyroid state after surgery gives signs of tetany and perioral paraesthesia. The presence of carpopedal spasm when the brachial artery is occluded, with a blood pressure cuff inflated above systolic blood pressure, is known as Trousseau's sign. Chvostek's sign involves tapping over the parotid gland and eliciting twitching of the facial muscles (this results from neuromuscular excitability).

A 46-year-old man with a history of bowel surgery presents with abdominal pain and vomiting. On examination there is some tenderness on palpation. Bowel sounds are tinkling. His abdominal radiograph shows dilated loops of small bowel.

G   Adhesions are fibrous bands that connect tissue surfaces that are normally separated. Formation of adhesions after bowel surgery can lead to bowel obstruction later. The patient may need to have another operation to cut the adhesions.

69 Haematuria

Answers: I L F G C

A 55-year-old smoker presents with painless haematuria and weight loss. Ultrasonography of the kidneys is normal.

I   Carcinoma of the bladder usually presents with total painless haematuria. Smoking and exposure to aniline dyes are risk factors for development of transitional cell carcinoma of the bladder. Treatment depends on the stage of disease. Most present with early disease that can be managed with diathermy. Other treatments include cystectomy, chemotherapy, radiotherapy and immunotherapy with intravesical BCG.
Carcinoma of the prostate usually presents with symptoms of poor stream, urinary obstruction and nocturia.

A 6-year-old boy presents with a 2-week history of non-blanching rash over the buttocks and macroscopic haematuria. He complains of pain in both knees.

L   Henoch–Schönlein purpura (HSP) usually occurs in young children and initially presents with a classic purpuric rash over the buttocks and extensor surfaces. Full blood count should reveal normal platelet count. There is joint involvement in around two-thirds of patients with the presence of periarticular oedema. Renal involvement is common with the presence of a focal segmental proliferative glomerulonephritis. IgA nephropathy may occur as a part of HSP. Abdominal pain is a common symptom and there is an increased incidence of intussusception in children with HSP. Children usually make a complete recovery.

A 9-year-old boy presents with periorbital oedema and microscopic haematuria plus proteinuria. ASOT is positive and serum C3 is reduced. Apart from a sore throat 2 weeks ago, he has no previous medical history of note.

F   Look out for the history of preceding pharyngitis, upper respiratory tract infection, etc., particularly in young men and children. There is a diffuse proliferative glomerulonephritis that is caused by the appearance of immune complexes after infection by group A β-haemolytic streptococci.

The prognosis in young children is excellent and renal biopsy is not usually necessary.

A 30-year-old man presents with a colicky loin pain that radiates to the groin area, which is associated with nausea and vomiting.

G   Renal calculi are more common in men. Risk factors include urinary tract infection, dehydration and conditions associated with hypercalcaemia. The pain of ureteric colic is severe and it is important to provide adequate analgesia for the patient.

A 75-year-old woman presents with frequency, pain on micturition and haematuria.

C   These are symptoms of acute cystitis. Acute pyelonephritis gives more severe symptoms of fever, rigors, vomiting and loin pain.

70 Weight loss

Answers: I C F G K

A 26-year-old woman complains of weight loss associated with diarrhoea and palpitations. Her pulse is irregular.

I   Thyrotoxicosis is a well-recognized cause of atrial fibrillation and so thyroid function tests should always be carried out on first presentation.

A 30-year-old Asian man complains of fever, weight loss, night sweats and persistent cough.

C   Haemoptysis may also occur and can be profound, e.g. cupfuls of blood. In the UK there is a much higher incidence of TB among immigrants from Asia and Africa than in the native population.

A 55-year-old woman presents with abdominal pain, weight loss and fatty stools. She also complains of extremely uncomfortable itchy blisters on her knees and elbows.

F   Coeliac disease is also known as gluten-sensitive enteropathy and is characterized by villous atrophy, giving rise to malabsorption in the small bowel; this reverses with a gluten-free diet. There is a particularly strong association with the HLA-DR3 and -DQ2 haplotypes. Dermatitis herpetiformis (DH) is an immune-complex-mediated (IgA) bullous skin disease that is associated with coeliac disease. DH can be treated with oral dapsone in the acute setting, but can usually be managed without medication by maintaining a gluten-free diet. Anti-endomysial antibodies have a high sensitivity and specificity for coeliac disease. Jejunal biopsy to detect villous atrophy, reversible on gluten removal from the diet, is the diagnostic investigation of choice.

A 10-year-old boy presents with a history of weight loss and excessive thirst.

G   Type 1 diabetes mellitus is usually of juvenile onset and is characterized by insulin deficiency. Common early symptoms include polydipsia, polyuria and weight loss. The patient may also present as a medical emergency with diabetic ketoacidosis. Signs of diabetic ketoacidosis include hyperventilation, dehydration, drowsiness, abdominal pain and vomiting.

A 24-year-old woman complains of tiredness and difficulty in concentrating at university. On examination she has marked weight loss and lanugo hair. Blood tests reveal a mild hypokalaemia.

K   Anorexia nervosa is characterized by a morbid fear of fatness and a desire to be thinner that is associated with a body mass index (BMI) less than $17.5\,kg/m^2$ (more than 15 per cent below standard weight). Lanugo hair is soft downy hair found particularly on the face and forearms, which is a feature of advanced anorexia. Hypokalaemia and alkalosis are sometimes found when blood tests are carried out to investigate weight loss, and result from self-induced vomiting and laxative and diuretic abuse.

71 Dysphagia

Answers: G I L K A

A 35-year-old woman presents with dysphagia for solid and liquids associated with regurgitation and weight loss. Barium swallow shows a dilated tapering oesophagus.

G   Oesophageal achalasia involves a failure of relaxation of the lower oesophageal sphincter on the initiation of swallowing. There are degenerative changes in both the myenteric plexus and the vagus nerve. It is important to perform a oesophagoscopy to exclude the possibility of carcinoma at the lower end of the oesophagus. First-line treatment involves endoscopic balloon dilatation of the sphincter. Surgical treatment involves dividing the muscle at the lower end of the oesophagus – known as a Heller's cardiomyotomy.

A 65-year-old smoker presents with a history of severe oesophagitis and gradually worsening dysphagia.

I   This history is highly suggestive of carcinoma. Smoking is a risk factor.

A 28-year-old woman presents with a feeling of a lump in her throat that causes some discomfort on swallowing. Examination and imaging of the pharynx and oesophagus reveal no abnormality.

L   Globus hystericus involves a classic description of a constant 'lump in my throat' sensation, but no abnormality can be found. Some patients describe a difficulty in swallowing whereas others claim that swallowing food/drinking liquids relieves the discomfort. The symptoms are often worse when the patient is feeling particularly stressed. It is important to rule out any other pathology before this diagnosis is made.

A 40-year-old man complains of intermittent dysphagia associated with chest pain. Barium swallow reveals a corkscrew oesophagus.

K   There is abnormal contraction of the oesophagus giving rise to the corkscrew appearance on barium swallow. Anti-spasmodics can be prescribed but are not always helpful.

A 55-year-old man presents coughing when he tries to swallow. On examination he has a flaccid fasciculating tongue.

A   There is difficulty in coordinating the swallowing movement. There is lower motor neuron weakness of the muscles supplied by the cranial nerve which lie in the medulla. The flaccid fasciculating tongue indicates nerve XII involvement.

72 Lower gastrointestinal bleeding

Answers: E L I J G

A 62-year-old man presents with rectal bleeding and a year's history of left iliac fossa pain and change in bowel habit. There is no weight loss.

E   Diverticular disease mainly occurs in the sigmoid colon. A high-fibre diet helps to prevent the high intraluminal pressures that are believed to cause diverticula.

An 8-month-old baby presents with inconsolable crying, colic and bleeding per rectum. A sausage-shaped abdominal mass is palpable.

L   Intussusception is a paediatric surgical emergency and refers to the invagination of proximal bowel into a distal segment. The most common pathology involves the ileum passing into the caecum and colon through the ileocaecal valve. This condition usually occurs in children between the age of 2 months and 2 years. Presentation is typically with inconsolable crying, colic (child classically draws the legs up) and a sausage-shaped mass in the abdomen. The rectal bleeding is sometimes described as having a redcurrant jelly-like appearance. The condition is usually treated by rectal air insufflation. If this fails, surgical intervention is indicated.

A 35-year-old man returns from holiday with a 2-week history of fever, cramping abdominal pain and bloody diarrhoea.

I   The acute history and recent travel history make infectious diarrhoea the most likely cause. Stool sample for microscopy, culture and sensitivity is the investigation of choice. If the patient is systemically unwell, anti-biotics (e.g. empirical treatment with ciprofloxacin) may be started before diagnosis is confirmed.

Common bacterial causes of dysentery include *Shigella*, *Campylobacter* and *Salmonella* spp. and *E. coli*.

A 60-year-old man complains of tiredness and significant weight loss. He notes episodes of rectal bleeding with blood mixed in with the stool over the last few weeks. There is no diarrhoea.

J   Colonic carcinoma should always be considered with a history of weight loss plus blood mixed in with the stool. However, right-sided lesions may present non-specifically with iron deficiency anaemia.
Risk factors include neoplastic polyps, inflammatory bowel disease (mainly ulcerative colitis) and a previous history of carcinoma. The 5-year survival rate of adenocarcinoma confined to the bowel wall is over 90 per cent and so surgery may be curative.

A 21-year-old man presents with a history of constipation and rectal bleeding. On examination there are numerous dark freckles on the palm, lips and oral mucosa.

G   This is a rare condition with the presence of polyps (hamartomas) that virtually never become malignant. Buccal pigmentation is an important sign.

73 Haematemesis

Answers: A B J E H

A 50-year-old man who is an alcoholic complains of vomiting blood. On examination he has signs of chronic liver disease.

A   Portal hypertension causes the diversion of blood through portosystemic anastomoses and the development of oesophageal varices. Alcoholic liver cirrhosis is by far the most common cause of oesophageal varices. The risk of rupture is particularly high if the patient is still drinking alcohol.

A 55-year-old businessman complains of epigastric pain worse at night, which is relieved by eating. He has started vomiting small amounts of blood.

B   Symptoms of duodenal ulcer are often relieved by eating, drinking milk, etc., whereas gastric ulcer symptoms are often aggravated by eating.

A 60-year-old woman with a several year history of heartburn presents with occasional haematemesis. Endoscopy reveals intestinal-type metaplasia at the distal oesophagus.

J   Barret's oesophagus is the term used to describe the presence of specialized intestinal metaplasia in the oesophagus (squamous to columnar) secondary to chronic reflux oesophagitis. There is an increased risk of developing adenocarcinoma of the oesophagus (40-fold increase is often quoted but the overall risk is still low).

Treatment involves the use of medication used to treat reflux oesophagitis (proton pump inhibitors, H_2-receptor antagonists, etc.) and also laser therapy to ablate intestinal metaplasia and allow regrowth of squamous epithelium.

A 40-year-old woman presents with haematemesis after a bout of prolonged vomiting.

E   A Mallory–Weiss tear is a mucosal tear at the gastro-oesophageal junction secondary to a sudden increase in pressure in that area usually mediated by a bout of severe coughing or vomiting. Alcohol binging and consequent vomiting are a major cause of Mallory–Weiss tear. Actively bleeding tears can be treated at endoscopy with electrocoagulation. Antiemetic therapy provides the mainstay of medical treatment.

A 60-year-old woman with pernicious anaemia presents with a 2-month history of dyspepsia, weight loss and haematemesis. Examination reveals an enlarged left supraclavicular node.

H   Pernicious anaemia (a condition characterized by atrophy of gastric mucosa and lack of intrinsic factor) is a risk factor for gastric carcinoma. Other risk factors include smoking and partial gastrectomy. An enlarged left supraclavicular node is known as a Virchow node and is an indicator of poor prognosis (Trousseau's sign).

74 Diarrhoea

Answers: H I F L J

A 19-year-old backpacker presents with a 2-day history of vomiting and watery diarrhoea.

H   Stool microscopy and culture is particularly important because the patient has recently been abroad.
Management should involve maintaining good oral fluid intake to replace fluids lost in diarrhoea and vomiting. Antibiotics are indicated if the patient is systemically unwell.

A 75-year-old patient treated with broad-spectrum antibiotics presents a few days later with bloody diarrhoea.

I   Pseudomembranous colitis (PMC) is caused by overgrowth of *Clostridium difficile* after antibiotic therapy. An important primary measure is to discontinue the suspected antibiotics because this can sometimes be sufficient to relieve symptoms. Metronidazole is the treatment of choice.

An anxious 31-year-old woman complains of a history of chronic diarrhoea alternating with constipation. She often feels bloated. Investigations are normal.

F   Irritable bowel syndrome is often more severe during times of stress. Some patients report relief of abdominal pain on passing flatus/defecation. Women are more frequently affected than men.

A 17-year-old man presents with symptoms of chronic diarrhoea and smelly stools. He has a history of recurrent chest infections as a child.

L   Cystic fibrosis can give rise to pancreatic insufficiency and consequently steatorrhoea caused by gastrointestinal malabsorption.

A 35-year-old woman with diabetes presents with weight loss, diarrhoea and angular stomatitis. Blood tests reveal presence of anti-gliadin antibodies.

J   Anti-endomysial antibodies (serum IgA) can also be used to diagnose coeliac disease and in fact show greater sensitivity and specificity. Jejunal biopsy shows villous atrophy, which is reversible on removal of gluten from the diet. There are general signs of malabsorption, e.g. folate deficiency macrocytic anaemia, excessive bleeding resulting from vitamin K malabsorption, etc. Coeliac disease is associated with an increased risk of developing gastrointestinal lymphoma.

75 Constipation

Answers: I J A K H

An 80-year-old woman presents with thirst, tiredness, depression, bone pain and constipation.

I   Hypercalcaemia is also a well-recognized cause of confusion. Intravenous saline, furosemide (frusemide) and bisphosphonates can be used to lower serum calcium.

A 65-year-old man presents with a 3-month history of weight loss, altered bowel habit and bleeding per rectum.

J   A patient with this history should be referred for colonoscopy as soon as possible.

A 42-year-old woman complains of weight gain, constipation, cold intolerance and depression.

A   Symptoms of hypothyroidism include cold intolerance, weight gain, hoarse voice, menorrhagia, constipation and depression.
On examination the patient may have the typical coarse facial features. Signs include bradycardia, goitre, non-pitting oedema, particularly over the eyelids, peripheral neuropathy and slowly relaxing reflexes. Hypothyroidism can also present as an emergency with confusion/coma (myxoedema coma). The patient may be hypothermic and hypoglycaemic and have chronic cardiac failure. Thyroid replacement therapy should be initiated gradually to prevent complications.

A 65-year-old woman presents with constipation and colicky left-sided abdominal pain relieved by defecation.

K   Diverticula are herniations of the gut wall (usually at the sigmoid colon) that probably result from high intraluminal pressures. Diverticular disease is far more prominent in western countries compared with those countries that adopt a diet containing more fibre. It is believed that a low-fibre diet contributes to raised intraluminal pressure and the development of diverticula. The incidence increases with age, such that about a third of the UK population will develop diverticula by the age of 65 years. The main complications to look out for are the development of inflammation (diverticulitis) and perforation. Remember that barium enema is contraindicated if diverticulitis is suspected (fever, raised C-reactive protein or CRP, raised white cell count, etc.) because of the risk of perforation.

A 21-year-old woman presenting with weakness and lethargy has been successfully treated for anaemia. She now complains of constipation and black stools.

H   Ferrous sulphate (iron tablets) is a common cause of constipation and black stools. Before embarking on invasive investigations it is important to ask about the drug history of the patient.

76   Abnormal abdominal radiographs

Answers: L G I A D

A 55 year old with a history of epigastric discomfort of several months presents acutely unwell in A&E. His radiograph shows free gas under the diaphragm.

L   Free gas under the diaphragm could result from any perforated viscus, e.g. colon and is not specific for gastric/duodenal perforation.

Abdominal film of an elderly constipated woman shows an 'inverted U' loop of bowel.

G   The sigmoid colon is the most common site of volvulus in the gastro-intestinal tract. The condition involves the sigmoid colon twisting around its mesenteric axis, causing obstruction. The condition tends to occur in elderly people. The condition can be treated by sigmoidoscopy and the insertion of a flatus tube per rectum to allow decompression.

A 31-year-old man presents with fever and bloody diarrhoea. He is tachycardic and has a Hb of 10.0 g/dl. Abdominal film shows loss of haustral pattern and a colonic dilatation of 8 cm.

I   This is toxic megacolon and a presentation of severe ulcerative colitis.

A 26-year-old student presents with bloody diarrhoea, abdominal pain and weight loss. Barium enema reveals 'cobble-stoning' and colonic strictures.

A   Strictures and fistulae are typical of Crohn's disease. Ulceration and fis-
       suring give rise to 'rose thorn' ulcers. There is discontinuous involvement
       of the gastrointestinal tract with skip lesions.

       **A 45-year-old man presents with severe epigastric pain and vomiting.
       Abdominal film shows absent psoas shadow and 'sentinel loop' of
       proximal jejunum.**

D   The absence of the psoas shadow is the result of a build up of retroperi-
       toneal fluid. The sentinel loop refers to a segment of gas-filled proximal
       jejunum. However, it is important to remember that an abdominal plain
       film can be completely normal in a patient presenting with acute
       pancreatitis.

77 Treatment of gastrointestinal conditions

Answers: E A J G H

       A 50-year-old man presenting with a perforated gastric ulcer.

E   This is a surgical emergency and requires laparotomy for surgical repair.

       **A 55-year-old woman with severe oesophagitis confirmed on
       endoscopy.**

A   High-dose proton pump inhibitor is indicated as first-line treatment to
       ensure healing. Once healed, low-dose therapy can be continued.

       A 60-year-old man with cirrhosis presenting with haematemesis.

J   Acute upper gastrointestinal bleeding is most commonly caused by
       peptic ulcer disease, except in patients with known cirrhosis when variceal
       bleeding is the cause in 85 per cent of cases. Suspected oesophageal
       varices are an indication for upper gastrointestinal endoscopy.

       **A 30-year-old man with ulcerative colitis presents to A&E with fever,
       tachycardia and abdominal distension.**

G   This is presentation of severe ulcerative colitis and intravenous
       hydrocortisone is indicated.
       Other markers of a severe attack are anaemia, marked rectal bleeding and
       an ESR significantly raised from baseline. When the patient improves
       after a few days, oral prednisolone and a maintenance agent such as
       sulfasalazine (sulphasazine) can be prescribed.

       **A 24-year-old woman with suspected irritable bowel syndrome
       complains of colicky pain and bloating.**

H   Mebeverine is an anti-spasmodic agent and relieves symptoms in some
       patients. This agent has the advantage of relaxing intestinal smooth
       muscle without anti-cholinergic side effects.

REVISION BOXES

The abdomen and surgery

EMQs describing abdominal pain are very common. Box 1 describes some classic presentations that you may find in questions.

Box 1 Abdominal pain [54, 55]

Classic presentation	Problem
Colicky loin pain radiating to groin	Ureteric colic
Jaundice and constant right upper quadrant pain	Biliary colic
Severe epigastric pain radiating to back associated with vomiting	Acute pancreatitis
Periumbilical pain radiating to right iliac fossa	Acute appendicitis
Central abdominal pain, expansile pulsatile mass	Abdominal aortic aneurysm
Iliac fossa pain, positive pregnancy test	Ectopic pregnancy

Box 2 summarizes various signs that may be mentioned in an EMQ which should prompt you to look for particular options in the question.

Box 2 On examination of the abdomen

Signs	Option
Asterixis (liver flap)	Hepatic encephalopathy
Leukonychia	Hypoalbuminaemia
Koilonychia	Iron-deficiency anaemia
Angular stomatitis	Iron-deficiency anaemia
Buccal pigmentation	Peutz–Jeghers syndrome
	Addison's disease
Glossitis	Vitamin B_{12} deficiency
Aphthous ulceration	Inflammatory bowel disease
	Coeliac disease
Expansile pulsatile mass	Aneurysm
Craggy hepatomegaly	Liver malignancy

Box 3 gives some examples of signs of liver disease particularly relevant to EMQs.

Box 3 Signs of chronic liver disease

Signs
Clubbing Flapping tremor Dupuytren's contracture Palmar erythema* Gynaecomastia Spider naevi* Splenomegaly* Testicular atrophy Ascites* Encephalopathy*

Signs	Condition
Chronic liver disease associated with: Early onset emphysema Pigmentation, diabetes Dysarthria, dyskinesia, dementia, Kayser–Fleischer ring	α_1-Antitrypsin deficiency [57] Haemochromatosis [57] Wilson's disease [57]
*Denotes signs that also occur in acute liver disease	

The two conditions primary biliary cirrhosis and primary sclerosing cholangitis are frequently confused with each other and commonly crop up in EMQs (Box 4).

Box 4 Differentiation of hepatobiliary conditions

Condition	Associated problems
Primary biliary cirrhosis [59]	Middle-aged woman presents with: Pruritus, jaundice, pigmentation Anti-mitochondrial antibody (AMA) positive

	Associated with: rheumatoid arthritis
	    Sjögren's syndrome
	    thyroid disease
	    keratoconjunctivitis sicca
	    renal tubular acidosis
	    membranous glomerulonephritis

Primary sclerosing cholangitis [59]	Usually middle-aged man, presents with: Pruritus, jaundice, abdominal pain $\uparrow$ ALP (alkaline phosphatase), AMA negative Associated with inflammatory bowel disease (especially ulcerative colitis)

Crohn's disease and ulcerative colitis are the two major forms of inflammatory bowel disease. There is significant overlap in the clinical features of these diseases.

Box 5 summarizes typical presentations and highlights differing features that are likely to be mentioned in EMQs.

Box 5 Features of inflammatory bowel disease (IBD)

IBD	Features
Crohn's disease [55, 76]	Can affect anywhere between mouth and anus Weight loss, diarrhoea, abdominal pain Strictures, anal fistulae Barium enema: 'cobble-stoning' 'Rose-thorn' ulcers Granulomas
Ulcerative colitis (UC) [76, 77]	Only affects colon Diarrhoea with blood and mucus Fever, tachycardia, toxic megacolon in severe acute UC Barium enema: loss of haustra Sigmoidoscopy: oedematous, friable mucosa

SECTION 7: METABOLIC AND ENDOCRINE DISTURBANCES

QUESTIONS

78 Endocrine problems

A	diabetes insipidus	H	diabetes mellitus
B	hyperparathyroidism	I	acromegaly
C	melanoma	J	syndrome of inappropriate
D	hyperprolactinaemia		ADH secretion (SIADH)
E	Nelson's syndrome	K	phaeochromocytoma
F	Cushing's disease	L	hypoparathyroidism
G	hyperthyroidism		

For each clinical scenario below, give the most likely cause for the clinical findings. Each option may be used only once.

1 A 40-year-old woman presents with skin hyperpigmentation after bilateral adrenalectomy.

2 A 21-year-old woman presents with amenorrhoea, vaginal dryness and galactorrhoea. On examination she has a bitemporal hemianopia.

3 A 26-year-old woman complains of weight gain, menstrual irregularity and hirsuitism. Examination reveals proximal muscle weakness and BP of 150/100 mmHg.

4 A 28-year-old woman presents with chest tightness and anxiety attacks. She is hypertensive and her ECG shows left ventricular hypertrophy.

5 A 40-year-old woman is worried about her changing appearance and deepening voice. On examination she has coarse oily skin, enlarged tongue and proximal muscle weakness. She also mentions paraesthesia in both hands of recent onset.

Answers: see page 203.

79 Nutritional deficiencies

A	thiamine	G	pyridoxine
B	vitamin D	H	copper
C	selenium	I	vitamin K
D	folic acid	J	vitamin B_{12}
E	vitamin C	K	nicotinic acid
F	vitamin A		

For each clinical scenario below, give the most likely cause for the clinical findings. Each option may be used only once.

1   A 30-year-old woman with poor diet complains of bleeding gums.

2   A 55 year old with alcohol problems presents with nystagmus, ophthalmoplegia and ataxia.

3   A 35-year-old patient recently diagnosed with coeliac disease complains of prolonged bleeding after a small cut. The prothrombin time is increased.

4   A 25-year-old African man presents with symmetrical dermatitis on sun-exposed skin, diarrhoea and depression. He has recently been on anti-TB treatment.

5   A 12-year-old boy presents with night-blindness.

Answers: see page 204.

80 Electrolyte and metabolic disturbances

A	hyperkalaemia	H	hypocalcaemia
B	hypomagnesaemia	I	selenium deficiency
C	hyperlipidaemia	J	hypercalcaemia
D	zinc deficiency	K	hypokalaemia
E	hypomanganesaemia	L	hypoglycaemia
F	hypernatraemia	M	hyperglycaemia
G	hyponatraemia		

For each clinical scenario below, suggest the most likely electrolyte/metabolic disturbance that is present in the patient in each question. Each option may be used only once.

1 A 40-year-old woman treated with spironolactone and lisinopril for heart failure presents with bradycardia. ECG shows tall, tented 't' waves.

2 A 30-year-old woman presents with tetany, perioral paraesthesia and carpopedal spasm after thyroid surgery.

3 A 30-year-old man being treated for a systemic fungal infection presents with muscle weakness, arrhythmias and tetany. His ECG shows prolonged P–R interval and prominent U waves.

4 A 50-year-old woman on total parenteral nutrition (TPN) presents with red crusted lesions around the nostrils and corner of the mouth.

5 A 45-year-old woman presents with thirst, abdominal pain and history of renal stones.

Answers: see page 205.

81   Disorders of sodium balance

A	low dietary intake	F	excessive sweating
B	diabetes insipidus	G	hypervolaemic hyponatraemia
C	nephrotic syndrome	H	insulin overload
D	Addison's disease	I	chronic liver disease
E	syndrome of inappropriate antidiuretic hormone (ADH) secretion	J	pseudohyponatraemia
		K	ACTH-secreting adenoma
		L	hyperosmolar non-ketotic coma

For each clinical scenario below, suggest the most likely cause for the disorder in sodium balance. Each option may be used only once.

1   A 55-year-old smoker presents with weight loss, haemoptysis and confusion. Urine osmolality 520 mosmol/kg and serum sodium 112 mmol/l.

2   A 30-year-old man presents with symptoms of polyuria and polydipsia. Plasma sodium 165 mmol/l, plasma osmolality 310 mosmol/kg, urine osmolality 190 mosmol/kg.

3   A 45-year-old man with type 2 diabetes mellitus presents with drowsiness and dehydration. Plasma sodium is 158 mmol/l and glucose 40 mmol/l.

4   A 50-year-old person with type 1 diabetes and hyperlipidaemia has a mild hyponatraemia. Plasma sodium 125 mmol/l.

5   Hyponatraemia associated with heavy proteinuria in a 55-year-old woman on long-term penicillamine treatment for rheumatoid arthritis.

Answers: see page 206.

82 Hypercalcaemia

A	sarcoidosis	H	vitamin D toxicity
B	secondary hyperparathyroidism	I	Paget's disease
C	venesection	J	benign hypocalciuric hypercal-
D	hypoparathyroidism		caemia
E	PTH-like hormone secretion	K	bone metastases
F	myeloma	L	thyrotoxicosis
G	tertiary hyperparathyroidism		

For each clinical scenario below, give the most likely cause for the hypercalcaemia. Each option may be used only once.

1   An 80-year-old woman presents with weight loss and back pain. Investigations reveal an elevated erythrocyte sedimentation rate (ESR) and marked excretion of immunoglobulin light chains in the urine.

2   A 35-year-old man presents with dry cough and shortness of breath. His chest radiograph shows bilateral hilar lymphadenopathy.

3   A 35-year-old woman with breast cancer complains of pain and tenderness over the upper lumbar region. Alkaline phosphatase 400 U/l.

4   A 55-year-old smoker has recently been diagnosed with squamous cell lung cancer. The bone scan is unremarkable.

5   Hypercalcaemia in a 45-year-old man after renal transplantation.

Answers: see page 207.

83 Diabetic complications

A	neuropathic arthropathy	H	diabetic jaundice
B	haemoglobinopathy	I	retinopathy
C	vascular arthropathy	J	pyoderma gangrenosum
D	amyotrophy	K	vasculitis
E	mononeuritis	L	autonomic neuropathy
F	rheumatoid arthritis	M	necrobiosis lipoidica
G	radiculopathy	N	peripheral neuropathy

For each clinical scenario below, suggest the particular diabetic complication that the patient is presenting with. Each option may be used only once.

1   A 50-year-old man with diabetes complains of impotence.

2   A 65-year-old man presents with loss of sensation in a stocking distribution.

3   A 45-year-old woman with diabetes presents with shiny areas on her skin with a yellowish colour and overlying telangiectasia.

4   A 50-year-old person with diabetes presents with a swollen joint with abnormal but painless movement.

5   An 85-year-old man presents with painful wasting of the quadriceps muscle of the right leg with absent knee reflex. The area is very tender.

Answers: see page 208.

84 Treatment of diabetes

A warfarin
B 0.9 per cent saline, intravenous insulin, metformin
C 0.9 per cent saline, intravenous insulin, potassium
D intravenous 5 per cent glucose
E 0.9 per cent saline, insulin, heparin
F rosiglitazone
G metformin
H lifestyle change
I 0.9 per cent saline, intravenous insulin and calcium gluconate
J tolbutamide
K intravenous 50 per cent glucose
L gliclazide
M oral glucose preparation

Choose, from the options above, the diabetic medication that is described/ indicated in the questions below. Each option may be used only once.

1 A 45-year-old man with type 2 diabetes presents with hyperglycaemic, hyper-osmolar, non-ketotic coma. Blood glucose 40 mmol/l.

2 First-line treatment for a 19 year old with diabetes and metabolic ketoacidosis.

3 A 25-year-old athlete with type I diabetes is brought to A&E. He is unconscious with a blood glucose level of 1.0 mmol/l.

4 A 21-year-old man with type 1 diabetes presents with dizziness. On examination he is alert and no abnormalities are detected. Blood glucose 2 mmol/l.

5 A 50-year-old man presents with symptoms of tiredness. Fasting glucose 6.8 mmol/l which rises to 10.7 mmol/l after oral glucose tolerance test.

Answers: see page 209.

ANSWERS

78 Endocrine problems

Answers: E D F K I

A 40-year-old woman presents with skin hyperpigmentation after bilateral adrenalectomy.

E   The removal of the adrenal glands has removed the physiological feedback inhibition of ACTH production. Excessive ACTH secretion gives rise to the increased pigmentation.

A 21-year-old woman presents with amenorrhoea, vaginal dryness and galactorrhoea. On examination she has a bitemporal hemianopia.

D   Symptoms of vaginal dryness, amenorrhoea and galactorrhoea are associated with hyperprolactinaemia. The presence of a bitemporal hemianopia suggests that the cause is oversecretion of prolactin by a prolactinoma. The treatment of choice is a resection via a transsphenoidal approach.
Drugs that have an anti-dopaminergic effect, e.g. metoclopramide and phenothiazines, can also cause hyperprolactinaemia.

A 26-year-old woman complains of weight gain, menstrual irregularity and hirsuitism. Examination reveals proximal muscle weakness and BP of 150/100 mmHg.

F   Cushing's syndrome is the term used to describe a state of glucocorticoid excess. This is usually caused by increased ACTH secretion from a pituitary tumour (Cushing's disease).
Other causes include ectopic secretion of ACTH by a tumour, e.g. small cell carcinoma, an iatrogenic excess of glucocorticosteroids and adrenal adenoma/carcinoma.
Some patients have a distinctive 'moon-shaped' face (although a cushingoid appearance can also be caused by excessive alcohol consumption) with a buffalo lump visible at the neck and centripetal obesity. The skin is usually thin and bruises easily with purple striae. There is a higher incidence of osteoporosis and pathological fractures.
Investigation aims to identify the cause. If plasma ACTH is very low/undetectable, the lesion is likely to be an adrenal tumour. The high-dose dexamethasone test can differentiate between ectopic ACTH/pituitary oversecretion if plasma ACTH proves to be detectable. An ectopic source of ACTH is associated with poor cortisol suppression, but a pituitary source (Cushing's disease) is associated with complete or at least partial suppression.

A 28-year-old woman presents with chest tightness and anxiety attacks. She is hypertensive and her ECG shows left ventricular hypertrophy.

K   Phaeochromocytoma is a tumour of the sympathetic nervous system that occurs in the adrenals in 90 per cent of cases. Ten per cent of phaeo-chromocytomas are malignant. Patients usually have evidence of significantly raised blood pressure and present with a range of symptoms, including headache, palpitations, chest tightness, blanching and anxiety attacks. Surgical excision is the treatment of choice.

A 40-year-old woman is worried about her changing appearance and deepening voice. On examination she has coarse oily skin, enlarged tongue and proximal muscle weakness. She also mentions paraesthesia in both hands of recent onset.

I   Acromegaly is caused by over-secretion of growth hormone (GH) from a pituitary adenoma. Most patients present with symptoms of change in appearance (particularly skin changes) or symptoms associated with mass effect of the tumour, e.g. headache, visual field defects. There are many changes in appearance caused by growth of soft tissues. Macroglossia and spade-like hands are particularly sensitive indicators of the presence of disease. Acromegaly is associated with hypertension, diabetes mellitus and cardiomyopathy with death usually occurring as a result of cardio-vascular pathology. The oral glucose tolerance test is diagnostic. Patients with acromegaly fail to suppress GH and indeed there may be a paradoxical rise in GH levels. Trans-sphenoidal surgical excision is the treatment of choice.

79 Nutritional deficiencies

Answers: E A I K F

A 30-year-old woman with poor diet complains of bleeding gums.

E   Vitamin C is involved in the hydroxylation of proline to hydroxyproline, which is necessary for the normal formation of collagen. In this scenario vitamin deficiency has led to scurvy.

A 55 year old with alcohol problems presents with nystagmus, ophthalmoplegia and ataxia.

A   This triad of symptoms is a sign of Wernicke's encephalopathy. Urgent thiamine is required to treat this condition to prevent progression to Korsakoff's syndrome. This is an irreversible condition characterized by anterograde and retrograde amnesia, resulting in confabulation.

A 35-year-old patient recently diagnosed with coeliac disease complains of prolonged bleeding after a small cut. The prothrombin time is increased.

I   Coeliac disease results in malabsorption of the fat-soluble vitamins (A, D, E, K). There are several vitamin K-dependent clotting factors (II, VII, IX, X) and so vitamin deficiency can lead to abnormal coagulation.

A 25-year-old African man presents with symmetrical dermatitis on sun-exposed skin, diarrhoea and depression. He has recently been on anti-TB treatment.

K   Isoniazid therapy can lead to nicotinic acid/vitamin B_6 deficiency. Pellagra is the name attributed to the symptoms of nicotinic acid deficiency. There is a predisposition to pellagra in patients with carcinoid syndrome because tryptophan metabolism is diverted away from nicotinamide production to produce amines.

A 12-year-old boy presents with night-blindness.

F   Vitamin A deficiency causes xerophthalmia with symptoms of night-blindness. Bitôt's spots are white areas of keratinized epithelial cells that can be seen in the conjunctivae of young children with vitamin A deficiency. Conjunctivae and corneas are typically dry and thickened.

80 Electrolyte and metabolic disturbances

Answers: A H K D J

A 40-year-old woman treated with spironolactone and lisinopril for heart failure presents with bradycardia. ECG shows tall, tented 't' waves.

A   There is significant risk of hyperkalaemia when spironolactone is co-prescribed with an angiotensin-converting enzyme (ACE) inhibitor. However, this combination is widely prescribed in the treatment of patients with moderate/severe heart failure because the addition of spironolactone to ACE inhibitor therapy was shown to improve survival in the RALES trial.

A 30-year-old woman presents with tetany, perioral paraesthesia and carpopedal spasm after thyroid surgery.

H   These are signs associated with hypocalcaemia resulting from inadvertent removal of parathyroid glands.

A 30-year-old man being treated for a systemic fungal infection presents with muscle weakness, arrhythmias and tetany. His ECG shows prolonged P–R interval and prominent U waves.

K   Hypokalaemia is a well-recognized adverse effect of amphotericin treatment secondary to increased renal loss. Flattened T waves and prominent U waves are ECG changes observed in hypokalaemia.

A 50-year-old woman on TPN presents with red crusted lesions around the nostrils and corner of the mouth.

D   Patients on TPN for a long period of time are at risk of becoming zinc deficient. Patients with zinc deficiency have these characteristic crusted lesions around the mouth and nostrils.

A 45-year-old woman presents with thirst, abdominal pain and history of renal stones.

J   There are numerous causes of hypercalcaemia, including malignancy, primary hyperparathyroidism, sarcoidosis and thyrotoxicosis. Initial management consists of aggressive rehydration with intravenous fluids. Further therapy is directed at treating the underlying cause where possible. Bisphosphonates are also useful in treating hypercalcaemia associated with malignancy. They act by inhibiting osteoclast resorption of bone and hence lower serum calcium levels.

81 Disorders of sodium balance

Answers: E B L J C

A 55-year-old smoker presents with weight loss, haemoptysis and confusion. Urine osmolality 520 mosmol/kg and serum sodium 112 mmol/l.

E   Syndrome of inappropriate ADH secretion (SIADH) is particularly associated with malignancy, especially small cell carcinoma of the lung. Other notable tumours include those of the central nervous system (CNS), prostate, pancreas, thymus and lymphomas. To make the diagnosis patients must be clinically euvolaemic with normal thyroid and adrenal function, a low plasma osmolality and inappropriately high urine osmolality.
        Other causes of SIADH include head injury, CNS disorders, e.g. meningoencephalitis, and metabolic disease, e.g. porphyria.
        Drugs that can cause SIADH include carbamazepine, chlorpropamide and cyclophosphamide.

A 30-year-old man presents with symptoms of polyuria and polydipsia. Plasma sodium 165 mmol/l, plasma osmolality 310 mosmol/kg, urine osmolality 190 mosmol/kg.

B   Diabetes insipidus (DI) is characterized by impaired water resorption by the kidney as a result of lack of ADH secretion by the posterior pituitary (cranial DI) or reduced sensitivity of the kidneys to the action of ADH (nephrogenic DI).
        Biochemistry reveals a high/borderline high plasma osmolality (patient always feels thirsty and tries to replace the lost fluid and lower plasma osmolality) with a low urine osmolality (the patient complains of production of large amounts of very dilute urine as a result of reduced water resorption in the kidney).

The water deprivation test is used to confirm diagnosis. A normal person will maintain his or her plasma osmolality and increase the urine osmolality (ADH working normally to maintain homoeostasis) in response to water deprivation. However, in a cranial DI patient there is a rise in plasma osmolality with production of dilute urine until exogenous ADH (vasopressin) is given.

In a nephrogenic DI patient the same plasma and urine osmolality changes occur but there is no response to the exogenous vasopressin.

A 45-year-old man with type 2 diabetes mellitus presents with drowsiness and dehydration. Plasma sodium is 158 mmol/l and glucose 40 mmol/l.

L Hyperosmolar non-ketotic coma (HONK) is a complication of type 2 diabetes. The patient usually has a history of poorly controlled diabetes or is undiagnosed before presentation. There is no acidosis. Appropriate first-line management of this patient would involve fluid replacement with 0.9 per cent saline. Insulin must be used with care because, if the plasma glucose falls too rapidly, there is a risk of a rapid change in osmolality causing cerebral oedema.

Anticoagulation is indicated as a result of the risk of thrombosis.

A 50-year-old person with type 1 diabetes and hyperlipidaemia has a mild hyponatraemia. Plasma sodium 125 mmol/l.

J Pseudohyponatraemia refers to a spuriously low plasma sodium concentration caused by hyperlipidaemia/hyperproteinaemia.

Hyponatraemia associated with heavy proteinuria in a 55-year-old woman on long-term penicillamine treatment for rheumatoid arthritis.

C In the nephrotic syndrome there is hypervolaemia, usually with clinically evident oedema, e.g. pedal oedema. Immune complex glomerulonephritis is common with penicillamine treatment and causes a mild proteinuria. The drug must be stopped but can often be resumed at a lower dose once the problem has resolved. However, heavy proteinuria is more serious and necessitates permanent withdrawal of treatment.

82 Hypercalcaemia

Answers: F A K E G

An 80-year-old woman presents with weight loss and back pain. Investigations reveal an elevated erythrocyte sedimentation rate (ESR) and marked excretion of immunoglobulin light chains in the urine.

F Even in the absence of the IgG chains in the urine, there are certain red flags here that suggest a sinister cause for the back pain, e.g. weight loss and elevated ESR. More than 1 g light chains excreted in the urine per day is a major criterion for the diagnosis of myeloma. Bisphosphonates may be used to treat hypercalcaemia associated with myeloma. Radiotherapy can be used to relieve bone pain.

A 35-year-old man presents with dry cough and shortness of breath. His chest radiograph shows bilateral hilar lymphadenopathy.

A   An abnormal incidental chest radiograph finding or respiratory symptoms are the initial presentations in up to 50 per cent of sarcoid patients. TB, malignancy, silicosis and extrinsic allergic alveolitis are other causes of bilateral hilar lymphadenopathy. There is a higher incidence of sarcoidosis among African–Caribbeans.

A 35-year-old woman with breast cancer complains of pain and tenderness over the upper lumbar region. Alkaline phosphatase 400 U/l.

K   Non-steroidal anti-inflammatory drugs (NSAIDs) such as ibuprofen are a particularly good first-line drug for the treatment of bone pain associated with metastases.

A 55-year-old smoker has recently been diagnosed with squamous cell lung cancer. The bone scan is unremarkable.

E   Ectopic parathyroid hormone (PTH)-related protein secretion by squamous cell carcinoma is a relatively rare cause of hypercalcaemia.

Hypercalcaemia in a 45-year-old man after renal transplantation.

G   Tertiary hyperparathyroidism involves the development of autonomous parathyroid hyperplasia that occurs after long-standing secondary hyperparathyroidism. Both plasma calcium and phosphate are raised. Secondary hyperparathyroidism is physiological hypertrophy of the parathyroid glands in response to hypocalcaemia. In this way, plasma calcium is usually low or normal in secondary hyperparathyroidism. Vitamin D deficiency and chronic renal failure are well-recognized causes of secondary hyperparathyroidism.

83 Diabetic complications

Answers: L N M A D

A 50-year-old man with diabetes complains of impotence.

L   Other signs include postural hypotension and urinary retention. Patients sometimes complain of diarrhoea that often occurs at night.

A 65-year-old man presents with loss of sensation in a stocking distribution.

N   This is the classic description of a peripheral neuropathy that always starts distally, hence the term 'glove-and-stocking' distribution.

A 45-year-old woman with diabetes presents with shiny areas on her skin with a yellowish colour and overlying telangiectasia.

M   Necrobiosis lipoidica most commonly appears over the shins. Pyoderma gangrenosum is not a diabetic complication and involves the presence of nodulopustular ulcers. It is associated with inflammatory bowel disease.

A 50-year-old person with diabetes presents with a swollen joint with abnormal but painless movement.

A   'Charcot's joints' is the term used to describe severe neuropathic arthropathy. Loss of pain sensation leaves swollen and deformed, yet painless, joints. Charcot's joints are also seen in syringomyelia and tabes dorsalis.

An 85-year-old man presents with painful wasting of the quadriceps muscle of the right leg with absent knee reflex. The area is very tender.

D   Diabetic amyotrophy is more common in the scenario of untreated diabetes in elderly people. It presents with a painful proximal motor neuropathy affecting the lower limbs. This is followed by weakness and wasting of the thigh muscles. The symptoms usually improve with good glycaemic control. This condition is distinct from the more common classic diabetic neuropathy.

84 Treatment of diabetes

Answers: E C K M H

A 45-year-old man with type 2 diabetes presents with hypergly-caemic, hyperosmolar, non-ketotic coma. Blood glucose 40 mmol/l.

E   Initial management of hyperosmolar, non-ketotic coma (HONK) involves treating the severe hyperglycaemia and dehydration that has occurred as a consequence of osmotic diuresis (occurs only in type 2 diabetes). It is associated with a high risk of thrombosis and hence heparin is indicated.

First-line treatment for a 19-year-old with diabetes and metabolic ketoacidosis.

C   Diabetic ketoacidosis is a medical emergency. Fluid replacement (with 0.9 per cent saline) is the most important initial measure. Hyperglycaemia should be treated with an intravenous infusion of insulin. This should be continued until ketones are absent from the urine. If the blood glucose falls to below 12 mmol/l during insulin infusion, 10 per cent glucose solution can be used for fluid replacement to buffer blood glucose until the insulin infusion can be discontinued. Patients usually present with hyperkalaemia caused by the metabolic acidosis. However, as a conse-quence of the prolonged osmotic diuresis preceding the acute presentation, they will have significant potassium depletion. As soon as insulin therapy has commenced, potassium levels will rapidly fall. Hence, patients will need regular potassium supplements in the intravenous fluids.

A 25-year-old athlete with type I diabetes is brought to A&E. He is unconscious with a blood glucose level of 1.0 mmol/l.

K   This is presentation of hypoglycaemic coma requiring immediate delivery of glucose. Oral glucose preparations are inappropriate in this acute situation as a result of risk of aspiration and should be given once the patient is conscious. In circumstances where intravenous glucose is difficult to administer, e.g. out of hospital, glucagon can be administered (subcutaneously, intramuscularly or intravenously).

A 21-year-old man with type 1 diabetes presents with dizziness. On examination he is alert and no abnormalities are detected. Blood glucose 2 mmol/l.

M   This patient has documented hypoglycaemia. Unlike the previous case he is conscious and relatively well. In this situation oral glucose solution is appropriate.

A 50-year-old man presents with symptoms of tiredness. Fasting glucose 6.8 mmol/l which rises to 10.7 mmol/l after oral glucose tolerance test.

H   This patient's test results suggest impaired glucose tolerance rather than frank diabetes. In both cases, lifestyle measures, e.g. diet control and weight reduction, are important.

REVISION BOXES

Metabolic and endocrine disturbances

Electrolyte imbalance can give rise to characteristic symptoms/signs. Calcium and potassium imbalance are the most common examples that are used in EMQs (Box 1).

Box 1 Symptoms/signs of metabolic disturbance [5, 6, 80]

Symptom/sign	Metabolic disturbance
• Cardiac arrhythmias ECG: tall 't' waves	Hyperkalaemia
• Muscle weakness, tetany ECG: small 't' waves, prominent U wave	Hypokalaemia
• Carpopedal spasm, perioral anaesthesia Positive Trousseau's, Chvostek's sign	Hypocalcaemia
• Many vague symptoms: Abdominal pain, constipation, vomiting Depression Anorexia (malignancy) Confusion (especially elderly people) Bone pain (malignancy) ↑ incidence renal stones ECG: reduced Q–T interval	Hypercalcaemia

Some vitamin deficiencies can give rise to well-defined symptoms/signs (Box 2).

Box 2 Signs of vitamin deficiency [79]

Signs	Deficiency
Prolonged bleeding	Vitamin K
Malnourished, bleeding gums (scurvy)	Vitamin C
Night-blindness	Vitamin A
Bowed legs (rickets)	Vitamin D
Nystagmus, ophthalmoplegia, ataxia	Vitamin B_1
Diarrhoea, dementia, dermatitis	Nicotinic acid
Sore red tongue	Vitamin B_{12} deficiency
Peripheral neuropathy	

Endocrine disturbance often gives rise to a plethora of symptoms and signs, the full details of which may be found in any good medical textbook.

The aim of Box 3 is to summarize some distinctive features of endocrine disease that commonly appear in EMQs.

Box 3 Endocrine disturbance [78]

Symptoms to look out for in questions:
- Heat intolerance, weight loss, diarrhoea, anxiety — Hyperthyroidism
- Cold intolerance, weight gain, depression, constipation, dementia, depression — Hypothyroidism
- Change in facial appearance, visual problems — Acromegaly
- Weight gain, hirsutism, menstrual problems, depression — Cushing's syndrome

On examination:
- Buccal/palmar crease hyperpigmentation, postural hypotension — Addison's disease
- 'Moon-shaped' face, centripetal obesity, proximal myopathy, purple striae, hypertension, diabetes mellitus — Cushing's disease
- Macroglossia, spade-like hands and feet — Acromegaly
- Bradycardia, dry thin hair, goitre, loss of outer third of eyebrow, slowly relaxing reflexes — Hypothyroidism
- Tachycardia, goitre, atrial fibrillation, lid lag — Hyperthyroidism

SECTION 8:
MISCELLANEOUS

QUESTIONS

85 Antibiotics

A   intravenous flucloxacillin plus
    benzylpenicillin
B   oral ciprofloxacin
C   oral gentamicin
D   intravenous cefuroxime plus
    metronidazole
E   intravenous gentamicin

F   oral rifampicin
G   oral tetracycline
H   intravenous vancomycin
I   oral nitrofurantoin
J   oral flucloxacillin
K   oral trimethoprim
L   oral/intravenous chloramphenicol

Choose, from the options above, the appropriate empirical therapy for the conditions below. Each option may be used only once.

1   A 35-year-old man with a hot swollen knee where septic arthritis is suspected.

2   A 54-year-old patient on the ward requires drug therapy for systemic methicillin-resistant *Staphylococcus aureus* (MRSA) infection.

3   A 23-year-old pregnant woman requires treatment for an uncomplicated urinary tract infection (UTI).

4   A 45-year-old woman requires antibiotic prophylaxis for a cholecystectomy.

5   A 25-year-old woman presents with sore throat and hoarseness of voice followed by pneumonia. Chlamydia serology is positive.

Answers: see page 230.

86 Antibiotics

A tetracycline
B cefuroxime + erythromycin
C tetracycline + chloramphenicol
D ceftriaxone
E flucloxacillin
F amoxicillin

G rifampicin
H teicoplanin
I ciprofloxacin
J nitrofurantoin
K isoniazid
L metronidazole

Choose, from the options above, the antibiotic therapy that is indicated for the presentations below. Each option may be used only once.

1 A 24-year-old woman complains of a yellow offensive vaginal discharge. Motile flagellate organisms are seen on wet film microscopy.

2 A 29-year-old man requires treatment for a severe community-acquired pneumonia.

3 A 25-year-old camper presents with fever, dehydration and severe bloody diarrhoea. Stool culture reveals salmonella infection.

4 An 18-year-old girl presents with fever, neck stiffness and photophobia.

5 A 24-year-old man presents with widespread impetigo over the face.

Answers: see page 231.

87 Treatment of infection

A	intravenous indinavir	G	topical malathion
B	intravenous fluconazole	H	foscarnet
C	intravenous amphotericin	I	flucytosine
D	intravenous malathion	J	oral terbinafine
E	intramuscular amphotericin	K	oral fluconazole
F	intravenous co-trimoxazole		

Choose, from the above options, the treatment that is indicated for the presentations below.

1   A 25-year-old man suffering from itchiness of hands and wrists. On examination burrows can be seen in the digital web spaces.

2   A 28-year-old man requires treatment for invasive aspergillosis.

3   First-line treatment for a 23-year-old woman complaining of vaginal itchiness and thick curd-like discharge.

4   A 45-year-old woman requires treatment for fungal toenail infections. She is on warfarin anticoagulation.

5   A 31-year-old HIV-positive man presents with pneumonia that began with a dry cough. His chest radiograph shows bilateral perihilar interstitial shadowing.

Answers: see page 231.

88 Antiviral therapies

A   aciclovir
B   amantadine
C   ribavirin
D   zidovudine, nevirapine,
    zanamivir
E   co-trimoxazole
F   AZT (zidovudine), didanosine,
    indinavir

G   interferon-β
H   ritonavir
I   zanamivir
J   ganciclovir
K   AZT, didanosine, ribavirin
L   interferon-α + ribavirin

Choose, from the options above, the antiviral agent(s) that is(are) indicated in the clinical situations below.

1   A 35-year-old man presents with a vesicular rash in a band over the umbilical area.

2   A 41-year-old HIV-positive man presents with decreased visual acuity. Fundoscopy shows a 'mozarrella and tomato pizza' appearance.

3   An infant is suffering from severe respiratory syncytial virus (RSV) bronchiolitis.

4   A 40-year-old man with chronic hepatitis C infection.

5   Highly active anti-retroviral therapy for a 28-year-old HIV-positive man.

Answers: see page 232.

89 Poisoning and overdose

A   captopril
B   atenolol
C   amitriptyline
D   heroin
E   ecstasy
F   paracetamol
G   cocaine

H   digoxin
I   diazepam
J   theophylline
K   aspirin
L   bendrofluazide
M   cyanide
N   carbon monoxide

Choose, from the above options, the drug that is responsible for each of the clinical presentations below. Each option may be used only once.

1   A 25 year old is rushed to A&E presenting with vomiting, hyperventilation, tinnitus and sweating. Blood gases show a respiratory alkalosis.

2   A man says that his depressed partner has taken an overdose. She is drowsy and hypotensive with signs of respiratory depression. There is no response to naloxone.

3   A 40-year-old depressed man is brought to A&E with dilated pupils, blurred vision and seizures. On examination he is tachycardic and his ECG shows wide QRS complexes.

4   A 35-year-old intravenous drug user (IVDU) presents comatose with pin-point pupils and respiratory depression.

5   A 42-year-old man presents with cyanosis and confusion. On examination he is noted to have the smell of almonds on his breath.

Answers: see page 233.

90 Treatment of poisoning and overdose

A	flumazenil	G	dicobalt edetate
B	desferrioxamine	H	atropine
C	*N*-acetylcysteine	I	atenolol
D	naloxone	J	intravenous fluids
E	dimercaprol	K	vitamin K
F	hyperbaric oxygen	L	metoclopramide + paracetamol

Choose the most appropriate pharmacological management for each of the presentations of poisoning/overdose below. Each option may be used only once.

1   A 40-year-old drowsy woman is brought to A&E with headache and vomiting with flushed cherry-pink skin. Carboxyhaemoglobin (COHb) is 40 per cent.

2   A 20-year-old woman presents to A&E with confusion, sweating and blurred vision after taking some ecstasy. She has a rectal temperature of 40.5°C. Creatine kinase is 4000 U/l.

3   A 32-year-old woman presents 6 hours after a paracetamol overdose. The paracetamol level is above the treatment line.

4   A 7-year-old boy presents to A&E with constricted pupils, sweating and increased salivation after drinking a bottle of insecticide lying in the garden.

5   A 54-year-old painter requires treatment for lead poisoning.

Answers: see page 234.

91 Adverse drug reactions

A	indinavir	H	adenosine
B	atropine	I	atenolol
C	simvastatin	J	zidovudine
D	nicotinic acid	K	captopril
E	cholestyramine	L	bendrofluazide
F	digoxin	M	lidocaine (lignocaine)
G	amiodarone	N	didanosine

Choose the medication that is giving rise to each of the presentations below. Each option may be used only once.

1   A 28-year-old man on anti-HIV therapy complains of circumoral paraesthesia.

2   A 55-year-old woman on treatment for ischaemic heart disease complains of muscle pains.

3   A 65-year-old woman with asthma complains of wheezing and shortness of breath after starting anti-hypertensive medication.

4   A 50-year-old woman on treatment for paroxysmal atrial fibrillation presents with a photosensitive rash.

5   A 55-year-old man on anti-hypertensive medication presents with gout.

Answers: see page 236.

92 Adverse drug reactions

A	insulin	H	ethambutol
B	rifampicin	I	isoniazid
C	pyridoxine	J	enalapril
D	bendrofluazide	K	glibenclamide
E	lithium	L	isosorbide mononitrate
F	amitriptyline	M	metformin
G	prednisolone	N	fluoxetine

Choose the medication that is giving rise to each of the presentations below. Each option may be used only once.

1   A 35-year-old woman presents with polyuria and polydipsia. She says that she is on medication for bipolar disorder.

2   A 25-year-old man on anti-TB therapy complains of orange discoloration of the urine.

3   A 56-year-old man complains of a persistent dry cough a few weeks after starting new anti-hypertensive medication.

4   A 50-year-old woman complains of a metallic taste in the mouth and anorexia after starting medication for her diabetes.

5   A 55-year-old woman presents with weight gain, hypertension and proximal myopathy.

Answers: see page 237.

93 Adverse drug reactions

A	methotrexate	H	atenolol
B	captopril	I	ethambutol
C	pyridoxine	J	nifedipine
D	isoniazid	K	salbutamol
E	spironolactone	L	beclomethasone
F	rifampicin	M	aminophylline
G	gold	N	penicillamine

Choose the medication that is giving rise to each of the presentations below. Each option may be used only once.

1   A 50-year-old man on treatment for heart failure develops gynaecomastia.

2   A 35-year-old woman being treated for tuberculosis presents with pain on eye movement and deterioration in vision.

3   A 45-year-old woman on long-term therapy for psoriasis presents with liver fibrosis.

4   A 65-year-old man complains of flushing, headache and ankle swelling after starting new medication for hypertension.

5   A 55-year-old man complains of cold hands and feet after starting new medication for his high blood pressure.

Answers: see page 238.

94 Adverse drug reactions

A   phenytoin
B   sumatriptan
C   phenelzine
D   chloroquine
E   gold
F   ibuprofen
G   sulfasalazine (sulphasalazine)
H   anti–TNF therapy

I   valproate
J   fluoxetine
K   phenobarbitone
L   cyclophosphamide
M   azathioprine
N   metoclopramide
O   lamotrigine

Choose the medication that gives rise to each of the presentations below. Each option may be used only once.

1   A 21-year-old woman treated with medication for migraine develops acute dystonia.

2   A 35-year-old man on treatment for depression complains of a severe throbbing headache soon after his evening meal. Blood pressure is markedly raised.

3   A 34-year-old woman suffers from haemorrhagic cystitis after receiving medication for systemic lupus erythematosus (SLE).

4   A 25-year-old man on treatment for seizures complains of acne and gum hypertrophy.

5   A 24-year-old woman on treatment for epilepsy is admitted with acute pancreatitis.

Answers: see page 239.

95 Adverse drug reactions

A	morphine	I	labetolol
B	lisinopril	J	isoniazid
C	chloramphenicol	K	streptomycin
D	ibuprofen	L	hydralazine
E	co-trimoxazole	M	penicillin
F	rifampicin	N	prednisolone
G	gentamicin	O	tetracycline
H	verapamil		

Choose the medication that is giving rise to each of the presentations below. Each option may be used only once.

1   A 32-year-old man on treatment for pulmonary TB presents with reduced sensation in a glove-and-stocking distribution.

2   A 65 year old develops a photosensitive rash after being prescribed an additional drug for hypertension. Antinuclear antibody test is positive.

3   A 72-year-old woman taking medication for osteoarthritis complains of dyspepsia.

4   A 68-year-old man complains of constipation after starting 'heart' medication.

5   A 55-year-old woman presents with a vertebral crush fracture.

Answers: see page 240.

96 Infections

A	*Clostridium difficile*	G	*Pneumocystis carnii*
B	*Salmonella* spp.	H	*Campylobacter jejuni*
C	*Treponema pallidum*	I	*Legionella pneumophila*
D	*Staphylococcus aureus*	J	*Clostridium perfringens*
E	*Coxiella burnetii*	K	*Neisseria meningitidis*
F	*Mycobacterium tuberculosis*	L	*Escherichia coli*

Choose the most likely infecting organism from the options above. Each option may be used only once.

1   A 10-year-old girl presents with fever, photophobia and neck stiffness.

2   A 40-year-old patient presents with bloody diarrhoea after treatment with broad-spectrum antibiotics.

3   A young man presents with progressive ascending weakness and areflexia in all four limbs a few weeks after a gastrointestinal infection.

4   A 33-year-old IVDU presents with fever, rigors and nightsweats. On examination he has a pansystolic murmur best heard at the lower sternal edge.

5   A 65-year-old woman presents with frequency and dysuria.

Answers: see page 241.

97 Infections

A	*Leptospira icterohaemorrhagiae*	G	*Clostridium perfringens*
B	*Proteus mirabilis*	H	*Coxiella burnetii*
C	*Brucella* sp.	I	*Mycobacterium tuberculosis*
D	*Chlamydia trachomatis*	J	*Salmonella* sp.
E	*Rickettsia akari*	K	herpes zoster
F	group A streptococci	L	*Pseudomonas aeruginosa*

Choose the most likely infecting organism from the options above. Each option may be used only once.

1   An 18-year-old young man with sickle-cell disease presents with osteomyelitis.

2   A 23-year-old Somali man presents with fever, nightsweats, weight loss and haemoptysis.

3   A 45-year-old man rescued from a mountaineering accident presents with an open fracture of the tibia. He is in severe pain and the lower left limb is cold and pulseless. The muscles of the distal limb are brownish-black in colour.

4   A 41-year-old sewer worker presents with fever, jaundice and reddened conjunctivae.

5   A 12-year-old boy presents a few days after a sore throat with a punctate, erythematous generalized rash that spares his face. He has a 'strawberry tongue'.

Answers: see page 242.

98 Medical emergencies

A   endotracheal intubation
B   Burr hole
C   100 per cent O_2, intravenous heparin
D   oral diazepam
E   tracheostomy
F   100 per cent O_2, intravenous diazepam
G   intravenous atropine
H   pericardiocentesis
I   100 per cent O_2, oral temazepam
J   non-invasive positive pressure ventilation
K   DC (direct current) cardioversion
L   intravenous dobutamine
M   cricothyroidotomy

Suggest the most appropriate emergency management from the options above. Each option may be used only once.

1   A 40 year old rescued from a factory fire presents with stridor and cyanosis. Endotracheal intubation is unsuccessful.

2   A 21-year-old man presents with status epilepticus.

3   A 35-year-old builder is brought to A&E after suffering a blow to the side of the head at work. He did not lose consciousness but 4 hours afterwards complained of a severe headache. He became very confused and his conscious level is deteriorating. On examination he has a dilated right pupil. Pulse 50 beats/min, BP 168/100 mmHg.

4   A 30-year-old woman is rushed to A&E after a stab wound to the chest. On examination her heart sounds are muffled and the jugular venous pressure (JVP) rises on inspiration. BP 75/40 mmHg.

5   A 34-year-old woman collapses at the airport arrivals lounge with sudden dyspnoea. BP 90/42 mmHg, Pao_2 6.0 kPa.

Answers: see page 244.

99 The confused patient

A	intravenous flucloxacillin	I	intravenous bendrofluazide
B	folic acid	J	intravenous fluids, insulin
C	fresh frozen plasma	K	oral prednisolone
D	subcutaneous insulin	L	Burr hole
E	triiodothyronine	M	intravenous thiamine, fluids
F	intravenous haloperidol	N	intravenous fluids, pamidronate
G	intravenous hydrocortisone	O	blood transfusion
H	intravenous fluids, propranolol		

Choose, from the above options, the most appropriate therapy that is indicated for the scenarios below. Each option may be used only once.

1   A 53-year-old man presents to A&E confused and unsteady on his feet. On examination he has nystagmus and bilateral lateral rectus palsies. He smells strongly of alcohol.

2   A 28-year-old woman presents confused and weak after collapsing in the street. Examination reveals tachycardia, marked hypotension and several depigmented patches over her body. Hb 14 g/dl, glucose 3.5 mmol/l, serum Na^+ 128 mmol/l, serum K^+ 5.4 mmol/l, serum Ca^{2+} 2.6 mmol/l.

3   A 15-year-old boy presents acutely confused with hyperventilation, vomiting and abdominal pain. Hb 14 g/dl, white cell count $13.0 \times 10^9/l$, glucose 19 mmol/l, platelets $160 \times 10^9/l$.

4   A 73-year-old woman with a history of metastatic breast cancer presents with vomiting and abdominal pain. She is found to be acutely confused. On examination positive findings include dry mucous membranes. Hb 10 g/dl, white cell count $7 \times 10^9/l$, glucose 4.5 mmol/l, platelets $350 \times 10^9/l$, corrected calcium 4.2 mmol/l, serum K^+ 3.5 mmol/l.

5   A 26-year-old woman presents with fever, confusion and agitation. Examination reveals an irregular pulse of rate about 240/min and the presence of a goitre.

Answers: see page 245.

100 Drugs and immunity

A	specific Ig	H	normal Ig
B	penicillamine	I	ciclosporin
C	TNF antagonist	J	botulism antitoxin
D	interferon-β	K	gold
E	tetanus immunization	L	methotrexate
F	interferon-α	M	rabies immunization
G	pertussis immunization		

Choose the therapy indicated for the clinical scenarios below from the above options. Each option may be used only once.

1   A 28-year-old man requires medication to prevent kidney transplant rejection.

2   A 35-year-old man reports being bitten by a bat while on holiday abroad a few weeks ago.

3   A 21-year-old man returning from a camping holiday presenting with diplopia and photophobia develops cardiorespiratory failure.

4   A 40-year-old woman with multiple sclerosis is prescribed medication to reduce the number of relapses.

5   A 30-year-old woman presents with a laceration on her hand sustained while gardening. She has not had any injections in the last 15 years.

Answers: see page 246.

ANSWERS

85 Antibiotics

Answers: A H I D G

A 35-year-old man with a hot swollen knee where septic arthritis is suspected.

A This is a medical emergency and urgent Gram staining and culture are indicated. *Staphylococcus aureus* is the most common infecting pathogen in septic arthritis. Intravenous benzylpenicillin plus flucloxacillin is the preferred treatment until sensitivities are known. Remember the possibility of opportunistic infection if the patient is immunocompromised, e.g. HIV positive.

A 54-year-old patient on the ward requires drug therapy for systemic MRSA infection.

H Vancomycin is a glycopeptide antibiotic and is indicated for the treatment of MRSA infection. It should be given only intravenously for systemic infection because it is not significantly absorbed when given orally. Teicoplanin is a similar glycopeptide antibiotic with a longer duration of action (so it can be given once daily).

A 23-year-old pregnant woman requires treatment for an uncomplicated urinary tract infection (UTI).

I Trimethoprim should not be given in pregnancy because it is a folic acid antagonist and teratogenic.
Quinolones and tetracycline should also be avoided. The adverse effects of nitrofurantoin include diarrhoea, vomiting, neuropathy and fibrosis. Nitrofurantoin should be avoided in pregnant mothers at term and in breast-feeding mothers.

A 45-year-old woman requires antibiotic prophylaxis for a cholecystectomy.

D Intravenous co-amoxiclav is an alternative prophylactic antibiotic regimen for abdominal surgery.

A 25-year-old woman presents with sore throat and hoarseness of voice followed by pneumonia. Chlamydia serology is positive.

G Tetracycline is first-line treatment for chlamydia infection. Tetracycline is absolutely contraindicated in pregnancy and when breast-feeding. Tetracyclines are deposited in growing bone and can lead to permanent staining of teeth and dental hypoplasia. Patients treated with tetracycline are told to avoid milk products because these decrease absorption of the drug.

86 Antibiotics

Answers: L B I D E

> A 24-year-old woman complains of a yellow offensive vaginal discharge. Motile flagellate organisms are seen on wet film microscopy.

I. This is a typical presentation of an infection with *Trichomonas vaginalis.* This protozoan pathogen is sexually transmitted, causing a vaginitis in women and a non-gonococcal urethritis in men. Successful management involves treating both the patient and the partner.

> A 29-year-old man requires treatment for a severe community-acquired pneumonia.

B   An intravenous combination of a broad-spectrum β-lactamase antibiotic, e.g. co-amoxiclav or a second-/third-generation cephalosporin, together with a macrolide, e.g. clarithromycin or erythromycin is the preferred empirical antibiotic choice for adults hospitalized with severe community-acquired pneumonia.

> A 25-year-old camper presents with fever, dehydration and severe bloody diarrhoea. Stool culture reveals salmonella infection.

I   Ciprofloxacin is indicated because this is a severe salmonella infection and the patient is systemically unwell.

> An 18-year-old girl presents with fever, neck stiffness and photophobia.

D   Intravenous benzylpenicillin can be used for meningococcal (*Neisseria meningitidis*) infections.

> A 24-year-old man presents with widespread impetigo over the face.

E   Impetigo is a highly infectious skin disease that is caused by *Staphylococcus aureus* infection in most cases. The typical lesion is a weeping, exudative area with a characteristic honey-coloured crusting on the surface. Topical fusidic acid can be used for small areas, but flucloxacillin is indicated if there is widespread impetigo.

87 Treatment of infection

Answers: G C K J F

> A 25-year-old man suffering from itchiness of hands and wrists. On examination burrows can be seen in the digital web spaces.

G   This is scabies infection and is treated topically with malathion. Topical 1 per cent lindane is also used to treat this condition. Both treatments are contraindicated in pregnancy.

> A 28-year-old man requires treatment for invasive aspergillosis.

C   Intravenous/liposomal amphotericin is the treatment of choice for invasive aspergillosis.

As a result of the risk of anaphylaxis, a small test dose of amphotericin should be given before the first infusion. Common adverse effects include nausea, vomiting, diarrhoea and headache. More severe adverse effects include hearing loss, diplopia, convulsions and peripheral neuropathy. Amphotericin is associated with renal toxicity and so it is important to monitor urea and electrolytes daily. Disturbances in renal function can lead to hypokalaemia (causing arrhythmias) and hypomagnesaemia.

First-line treatment for a 23-year-old woman complaining of vaginal itchiness and thick curd-like discharge.

K   This is a presentation of vulvovaginal candidiasis, commonly referred to as thrush. Medical treatment can be topical with the use of azole pessaries/creams. Alternatively, single dose oral treatment with a triazole, e.g. fluconazole, can be used.

A 45-year-old woman requires treatment for fungal toenail infections. She is on warfarin anticoagulation.

J   Oral terbinafine is the treatment of choice for the systemic treatment of onychomycosis. The azoles are cytochrome P450 enzyme inhibitors and so their use could result in enhanced toxicity of warfarin (which is metabolized by cytochrome P450 enzymes).

Griseofulvin can also be used for the treatment of nail infections. It is a cytochrome P450 enzyme inducer and therefore its use would reduce the level of anticoagulation provided by the warfarin dose. The precipitation/aggravation of systemic lupus erythematosus (SLE) is a rare but well-recognized adverse effect of griseofulvin treatment.

A 31-year-old HIV-positive man presents with pneumonia that began with a dry cough. His chest radiograph shows bilateral perihilar interstitial shadowing.

F   This is the presentation of *Pneumocystis carinii* pneumonia (PCP). Co-trimoxazole is a combination of one part trimethoprim to five parts sulfamethoxazole. The sulphonamide component is associated with several adverse reactions, e.g. Stevens–Johnson syndrome and blood dyscrasias. Therefore, such combination therapy is restricted to conditions such as PCP where the synergistic activity merits its use.

The use of corticosteroids has been shown to be of some benefit in the treatment of PCP when the patient is hypoxaemic ($Pao_2 < 9.3$ kPa).

88 Antiviral therapies

Answers: A J C L F

A 35-year-old man presents with a vesicular rash in a band over the umbilical area.

A   This is a herpes zoster infection (shingles). Oral aciclovir is the treatment
        of choice.

        **A 41-year-old HIV-positive man presents with decreased visual acuity.
        Fundoscopy shows a 'mozarrella and tomato pizza' appearance.**

J   Cytomegalovirus (CMV) retinitis usually occurs only when the CD4 count
        has dropped to below 100. The diagnosis is made clinically. Fundoscopy
        reveals a characteristic 'pizza' appearance caused by the appearance of
        haemorrhages and exudates that follow the retinal vessels.
        CMV retinitis is a medical emergency as a result of the risk of blindness
        and should be treated with intravenous ganciclovir. Foscarnet can also
        be used to treat CMV retinitis.

        **An infant is suffering from severe respiratory syncytial virus (RSV)
        bronchiolitis.**

C   Inhaled ribavirin is indicated, although there is not yet clear evidence
        that it provides significant clinical benefit. A monoclonal antibody is
        now available that can be used to prevent RSV infection in infants at
        high risk (palivizumab).

        A 40-year-old man with chronic hepatitis C infection.

L   Interferon-α is given by subcutaneous injection. Combination therapy
        with ribavirin is more effective and should be continued for 6 months.

        **Highly active anti-retroviral therapy for a 28-year-old
        HIV-positive man.**

F   AZT, didanosine and indinavir provide a combination of two nucleoside
        sanalogue reverse transcriptase inhibitors (AZT, didanosine) with one pro-
        tease inhibitor (indinavir), which is commonly referred to as highly active
        anti-retroviral therapy (HAART). Non-nucleoside analogue reverse tran-
        scriptase inhibitors, e.g. nevirapine, can also be used as part of HAART.

89 Poisoning and overdose

Answers: **K I C D M**

        **A 25 year old is rushed to A&E presenting with vomiting,
        hyperventilation, tinnitus and sweating. Blood gases show a
        respiratory alkalosis.**

K   Patients initially present with a respiratory alkalosis caused by
        hyperventilation (stimulation of the respiratory centre) but a metabolic
        acidosis may develop later.
        Multiple doses of oral activated charcoal reduces the absorption of
        aspirin and is more effective the earlier it is given.
        Management of overdose can be classified according to
        mild/moderate/severe overdose.

If the salicylate concentration is below 500 mg/l in an adult or 350 mg/l in a child and there is no acidosis, then observations, fluids and symptomatic support are usually sufficient.

If salicylate concentration is above 500 mg/l in an adult or 350 mg/l in a child, alkaline diuresis with intravenous sodium bicarbonate is indicated. Forced diuresis is no longer used because it can cause cerebral and pulmonary oedema.

If the overdose is severe (salicylate concentration exceeds 700 mg/l), haemodialysis is indicated.

A man says that his depressed partner has taken an overdose. She is drowsy and hypotensive with signs of respiratory depression. There is no response to naloxone.

I   Toxicity is enhanced when benzodiazepines are taken with alcohol or other drugs.

A 40-year-old depressed man is brought to A&E with dilated pupils, blurred vision and seizures. On examination he is tachycardic and his ECG shows wide QRS complexes.

C   Amitriptyline is a tricyclic antidepressant. Anticholinergic effects are seen in overdose, e.g. dry mouth, dilated pupils, urinary retention and tachycardia. The presence of arrhythmias indicates cardiotoxicity but the use of anti-arrhythmic therapy is often not beneficial. The use of sodium bicarbonate is indicated to correct any associated acidosis.

A 35-year-old IVDU presents comatose with pin-point pupils and respiratory depression.

D   Remember that cocaine, amphetamine and tricyclics dilate the pupil but heroin constricts it. Heroin overdose is treated with naloxone (a competitive opioid receptor antagonist).

A 42-year-old man presents with cyanosis and confusion. On examination he is noted to have the smell of almonds on his breath.

M   Intravenous dicobalt edetate is the antidote of choice for cyanide poisoning. Other antidotes include intravenous hydroxycobalamin or combination treatment with sodium nitrite followed by sodium thiosulphate.

90 Treatment of poisoning and overdose

Answers: F J C H E

A 40-year-old drowsy woman is brought to A&E with headache and vomiting with flushed cherry-pink skin. Carboxyhaemoglobin (COHb) is 40 per cent.

F   This is a presentation of severe carbon monoxide poisoning, so hyperbaric oxygen therapy is indicated.

A 20-year-old woman presents to A&E with confusion, sweating and blurred vision after taking some ecstasy. She has a rectal temperature of 40.5°C. Creatine kinase (CK) is 4000 U/l.

J   The patient is hyperthermic and should be immediately transferred to intensive care for active cooling and fluid replacement (via central line).

A 32-year-old woman presents 6 hours after a paracetamol overdose. The paracetamol level is above the treatment line.

C   The metabolism of paracetamol involves the conversion to the toxic metabolite *N*-acetyl-*p*-benzoquinonimine (NAPQI), which covalently binds with sulphydryl groups on liver cell membranes, leading to liver cell necrosis. NAPQI generated by safe doses of paracetamol is normally inactivated by reduction with glutathione. However, large doses of paracetamol deplete glutathione stores, leading to toxic levels of NAPQI and hence hepatocellular damage.
N-Acetylcysteine and oral methionine are sulphydryl donors that act as precursors to glutathione, and hence help to replenish depleted glutathione stores.

A 7-year-old boy presents to A&E with constricted pupils, sweating and increased salivation after drinking a bottle of insecticide lying in the garden.

H   Organophosphate insecticides are cholinesterase inhibitors and therefore poisoning results in an accumulation of acetylcholine (muscarinic and nicotinic acetylcholine receptor activation). Any contaminated skin should be washed (wear gloves during all contact with the patient, e.g. removing patient's clothes). Medical first-line treatment involves intravenous atropine until full atropinization (i.e. patient has dilated pupils, flushed dry skin, heart rate normalized). Pralidoxime mesilate (cholinesterase activator) by slow intravenous injection is used as an adjunct to atropine.

A 54-year-old painter requires treatment for lead poisoning.

E   Chronic lead poisoning was more common when water pipes were made of lead. Lead poisoning is now more commonly occupational, e.g. exposure to lead-based paints, metal workers. Lead poisoning affects many organs as a result of its interference with enzyme systems and so presentation can involve many non-specific symptoms/signs. These include nausea, vomiting, abdominal pain, anaemia, constipation and sleep disturbance. There are no pathognomonic signs but a characteristic sign in children is the appearance of dense metaphyseal bands indicating arrested growth on a radiograph. These are known as lead lines.
Calcium EDTA and D-penicillamine have also been used in the treatment of lead poisoning by acting as chelators. Incidentally, dimercaprol is also used to treat other types of heavy metal poisoning, e.g. arsenic, mercury.

91 Adverse drug reactions

Answers: A C I G L

> **A 28-year-old man on anti-HIV therapy complains of circumoral paraesthesia.**

A   Adverse effects of the protease inhibitors also include fat redistribution (e.g. buffalo hump) and metabolic disturbances, e.g. glucose intolerance and hypertriglyceridaemia. Most protease inhibitors are cytochrome P450 inhibitors and therefore drug toxicity of other medications is possible.

> **A 55-year-old woman on treatment for ischaemic heart disease complains of muscle pains.**

C   The presence of muscle pain is not a contraindication to continuing therapy. The presence of myositis, on the other hand, which is inflammation of the muscle associated with markedly elevated CK levels, merits immediate discontinuation of treatment.
There is an increased risk of myopathy if a patient is taking a statin plus a fibrate drug, and so close monitoring of CK levels is particularly relevant in this group of individuals. Liver function tests should be carried out before starting treatment, a month/2 months after initiating treatment and then repeated every 6 months. Serum transaminase levels of above around three times the reference range are an indication to stop treatment.

> **A 65-year-old woman with asthma complains of wheezing and shortness of breath after starting anti-hypertensive medication.**

I   All β blockers are contraindicated in patients with asthma, even those that are β_1 selective.

> **A 50-year-old woman on treatment for paroxysmal atrial fibrillation presents with a photosensitive rash.**

G   Patients should be advised to avoid exposure to direct sunlight because of photosensitivity.
Corneal microdeposits occur in most patients and regress on termination of the treatment. They rarely affect visual acuity, but some patients may be dazzled by headlights at night.
Thyroid function tests should be carried out before treatment and every 6 months after starting treatment because amiodarone can cause hypo-/hyperthyroidism. This is usually reversible on withdrawal of treatment.

> **A 55-year-old man on anti-hypertensive medication presents with gout.**

L   Thiazide diuretics reduce renal excretion of uric acid, thus increasing plasma urate levels which may precipitate gout.

92 Adverse drug reactions

Answers: E B J M G

> A 35-year-old woman presents with polyuria and polydipsia. She says that she is on medication for bipolar disorder.

E   Polyuria and polydipsia are suggestive of diabetes insipidus. Lithium is a well-recognized drug cause of nephrogenic diabetes insipidus. Lithium has a narrow therapeutic window and so therapeutic drug monitoring is very important. Signs of toxicity include tremor, ataxia and dysarthria.

> A 25-year-old man on anti-TB therapy complains of orange discoloration of the urine.

B   Rifampicin can cause bodily secretions, such as saliva, tears and urine, to be coloured orange–red. Rifampicin is a potent cytochrome P450 inducer and thus has the potential to reduce plasma levels of cytochrome P450 substrates. If a drug is prescribed with rifampicin, the dose needs to be increased to compensate.

> A 56-year-old man complains of a persistent dry cough a few weeks after starting new anti-hypertensive medication.

J   Angiotensin-converting enzyme (ACE) (also known as kininase II) converts inactive angiotensin I to the vasoconstrictor angiotensin II. In this way, ACE inhibitors reduce angiotensin II levels.
     ACE also inactivates bradykinin and so ACE inhibitors may cause a persistent dry cough resulting from increased levels of bradykinin.

> A 50-year-old woman complains of a metallic taste in the mouth and anorexia after starting medication for her diabetes.

M   Metformin is particularly useful in treating overweight patients with type 2 diabetes mellitus because of its anorectic effect (sulphonylureas can encourage weight gain). Metformin reduces glucose absorption from the gut, inhibits liver gluconeogenesis and increases uptake of glucose into tissues. Hypoglycaemia does not usually occur with metformin treatment. Lactic acidosis is a very rare complication of metformin treatment but carries a high mortality. Metformin is therefore contraindicated in patients who are at risk of lactic acidosis, e.g. significant renal impairment. Metformin should be replaced with insulin before elective surgery.

> A 55-year-old woman presents with weight gain, hypertension and proximal myopathy.

G   The use of corticosteroids can give rise to an iatrogenic Cushing's syndrome. Therefore, long-term adverse effects of steroid treatment include diabetes, osteoporosis and hypertension.

93 Adverse drug reactions

Answers: E I A J H

> **A 50-year-old man on treatment for heart failure develops gynaecomastia.**

E
Spironolactone has a similar structure to aldosterone and functions as an aldosterone antagonist. Gynaecomastia is a recognized adverse effect caused by the action of spironolactone on sex hormone receptors. Gynaecomastia is also a recognized adverse effect of digoxin therapy. As spironolactone is a potassium-sparing diuretic, there is a risk of hyperkalaemia if it is given alongside an ACE inhibitor. Nevertheless, the addition of low-dose spironolactone therapy in patients with moderate/severe heart failure who are being treated with an ACE inhibitor has been shown to improve survival (see Question 8, p. 19).

> **A 35-year-old woman being treated for tuberculosis presents with pain on eye movement and deterioration in vision.**

I
Optic neuritis is an adverse effect of ethambutol treatment, giving rise to a painful eye and defective central vision. Visual acuity should be tested before treatment. Remember that the patient suffering from these symptoms/signs may have a normal optic disc on fundoscopic examination as he or she may be suffering from retrobulbar neuritis.

> **A 45-year-old woman on long-term therapy for psoriasis presents with liver fibrosis.**

A
Methotrexate is prescribed only when the patient has severe psoriasis that is resistant to other initial pharmacological therapy. Pulmonary fibrosis and hepatic fibrosis are recognized adverse effects of methotrexate treatment. Patients need to have a full blood count and tests for liver and renal function before treatment is started. These tests should be carried out regularly (e.g. weekly) while the treatment is being stabilized and then every 3 months thereafter.
As methotrexate is an anti-folate drug, it is considered teratogenic, so women should be counselled about the need to discontinue treatment for several months before conceiving.

> **A 65-year-old man complains of flushing, headache and ankle swelling after starting new medication for hypertension.**

J
Nifedipine is a voltage-dependent Ca^{2+} channel blocker. The flushing and headache are related to the arteriolar vasodilatation caused by nifedipine. Ankle swelling is caused by lymphatic paralysis and so does not respond very well to diuretics.

> **A 55-year-old man complains of cold hands and feet after starting new medication for his high blood pressure.**

H β-Adrenoceptor receptor blockade by a β-adrenoceptor antagonist (β blocker) can cause symptoms of cold peripheries and impotence, which may affect compliance. All β-adrenoceptor antagonists are contraindicated in patients with asthma as a result of the risk of airway obstruction.

β Blockers have a role in many aspects of cardiovascular disease, including treatment of hypertension, angina and arrhythmias.

β Blockers can also be used under specialist control for the treatment of heart failure.

94 Adverse drug reactions

Answers: N C L A I

A 21-year-old woman treated with medication for migraine develops acute dystonia.

N Acute dystonic reactions (including oculogyric crises) are recognized adverse effects of metoclopramide. These reactions are more common in the young.

Metoclopramide is a dopamine receptor antagonist that acts centrally on the chemoreceptor trigger zone (CTZ). It also acts directly on the gastrointestinal tract to prevent vomiting by enhancing gastric emptying.

A 35-year-old man on treatment for depression complains of a severe throbbing headache soon after his evening meal. Blood pressure is markedly raised.

C This is a presentation of a 'cheese' reaction. Many foods, e.g. cheese and yeast products, contain tyramine which is normally metabolized by monoamine oxidases in the gut wall and liver. However, phenelzine is a monoamine oxidase inhibitor and thus allows a larger amount of tyramine to reach the systemic circulation. Tyramine is a sympathomimetic and, therefore, the potentiation of this action by monoamine oxidase inhibition can give rise to an acute hypertensive crisis. The treatment of choice is intravenous phentolamine (α-adrenoceptor antagonist).

Reversible monoamine oxidases (reversibly inhibit monoamine oxidase type A) are available, e.g. meclobemide, which are claimed to cause less potentiation of the tyramine effect. However, patients should be counselled very carefully regarding the avoidance of tyramine-rich food when prescribed either class of drug.

A 34-year-old woman suffers from haemorrhagic cystitis after receiving medication for systemic lupus erythematosus (SLE).

L Cyclophosphamide is a potent cytotoxic drug that can be used to induce remission of severe flares of SLE.

When cyclophosphamide is broken down, its toxic metabolites (e.g. acrolein), which are irritant to the lining of the urinary tract, give rise to a haemorrhagic cystitis. Mesna is a drug that is prescribed with cyclophosphamide to protect the uroepithelium. It acts by inhibiting the decomposition of intermediate metabolites to acrolein and also binds directly with acrolein to prevent its toxic effect.

A 25-year-old man on treatment for seizures complains of acne and gum hypertrophy.

A Acne, gum hypertrophy, nausea, vomiting and tremor are all recognized adverse effects of phenytoin treatment. Blurred vision, ataxia or peripheral neuropathy are signs of drug toxicity. Phenytoin has a narrow therapeutic index and toxicity may easily occur.
Adjustment of dose of phenytoin is complicated by the fact that it has zero-order kinetics. This means that relatively small increases in dose can give rise to large increases in plasma concentration and consequently toxicity.

A 24-year-old woman on treatment for epilepsy is admitted with acute pancreatitis.

I Acute pancreatitis is a rare adverse effect of valproate therapy but patients should be informed of the symptoms and advised to seek immediate medical attention if these develop.

95 Adverse drug reactions

Answers: J L D H N

A 32-year-old man on treatment for pulmonary TB presents with reduced sensation in a glove-and-stocking distribution.

J Isoniazid is metabolized in the liver by acetylation. Toxicity in the form of peripheral neuropathy is more common in patients with a slow acetylator status, whereas fast acetylators are more likely to suffer from an isoniazid-related hepatitis. Rapid acetylator status is extremely common in the Japanese population (over 90 per cent). In the European population slow acetylator status is slightly more common (55–60 per cent).
This is an example of a genetic polymorphism affecting drug metabolism and toxicity.
Sensitivity to ethanol and suxamethonium are other examples of variations in drug metabolism caused by genetic polymorphism.

A 65 year old develops a photosensitive rash after being prescribed an additional drug for hypertension. Antinuclear antibody test is positive.

L An SLE-like syndrome with a positive antinuclear antibody test can be caused by a number of drugs, including hydralazine, procainamide, isoniazid, griseofulvin, chlorpromazine and anticonvulsants. The symptoms usually disappear on removal of the drug.

A 72-year-old woman taking medication for osteoarthritis complains of dyspepsia.

D   Dyspepsia is common with non-steroidal anti-inflammatory drugs (NSAIDs) because they block the production of gastro-protective prostaglandins in the stomach.

There is little evidence that NSAIDs provide a significantly superior analgesic effect to paracetamol in the management of osteoarthritic pain.

A 68-year-old man complains of constipation after starting 'heart' medication.

H   Verapamil is a calcium channel antagonist and constipation can result from the effect of blocking calcium channels in the gastrointestinal smooth muscle.

It is used in the treatment of supraventricular arrhythmias (class IV anti-arrhythmic drugs), e.g. prophylaxis of recurrent supraventricular tachycardia. It can also be used as rate control in patients with atrial fibrillation that is poorly controlled with digoxin alone.

Verapamil can be used in the treatment of hypertension and angina but should be avoided in heart failure because it reduces cardiac output.

A 55-year-old woman presents with a vertebral crush fracture.

N   Long-term corticosteroid therapy can predispose to osteoporosis and thus pathological fractures. The pathological state of osteoporosis is not associated with pain; it is the fracture that results from the loss of bone density that causes pain. The lumbar vertebrae, distal radius and femoral neck are the classic sites of osteoporotic fracture.

96 Infections

Answers: K A H D L

A 10-year-old girl presents with fever, photophobia and neck stiffness.

K   These symptoms and signs are suggestive of meningitis, most likely to be meningococcal/pneumococcal infection. This is a medical emergency and antibiotic therapy must be commenced immediately and without delay. Cerebrospinal fluid (CSF) analysis of a typical bacterial meningitis shows a very high neutrophil count, glucose less than half of the plasma value and increased protein.

A 40-year-old patient presents with bloody diarrhoea after treatment with broad-spectrum antibiotics.

A   This is a presentation of pseudomembranous colitis (PMC) and is caused by overgrowth of *Clostridium difficile*. The symptoms result from the toxins produced by the organism. Sigmoidoscopy usually reveals the characteristic erythematous and ulcerated mucosa covered by

pseudomembranes, but in a proportion of patients the site of disease is more proximal and would therefore not be detected.
Diagnosis is confirmed by detection of the toxin in the stool.

A young man presents with progressive ascending weakness and areflexia in all four limbs a few weeks after a gastrointestinal infection.

H   This is presentation of Guillain–Barré syndrome. There is a recognized association between a preceding gastrointestinal infection and the development of this condition. Around 70–85 per cent of patients make a complete/almost complete recovery. The most important complication of Guillain–Barré syndrome is the involvement of respiratory muscles. Arterial blood gases and bedside spirometry (forced vital capacity) should be monitored daily to detect significant compromise early.
High-dose intravenous immunoglobulin can reduce the severity and duration of illness in some patients.

A 33-year-old IVDU presents with fever, rigors and nightsweats. On examination he has a pansystolic murmur best heard at the lower sternal edge.

D   This is the presentation of infective endocarditis. The signs suggest that there is tricuspid valve involvement. Right-sided endocarditis occurs more commonly in intravenous drug users where *Staphylococcus aureus* is the most common infecting organism. In others, a large variety of organisms may cause bacterial endocarditis including α-haemolytic streptococci and more rarely the HACEK group (*Haemophilus, Actinobacillus, Cardiobacterium, Eikenella, Kingella*).

A 65-year-old woman presents with frequency and dysuria.

L   *E. coli* is the most common cause of urinary tract infection. *Klebsiella* sp. and *Proteus mirabilis* are other common pathogens.

97 Infections

Answers: J I G A F

An 18-year-old young man with sickle-cell disease presents with osteomyelitis.

J   *Staphylococcus aureus* infection is by far the most common infecting organism in acute osteomyelitis. It is important to remember that *Salmonella* sp. infection is a well-recognized cause of osteomyelitis in a patient with sickle-cell disease.

A 23-year-old Somali man presents with fever, nightsweats, weight loss and haemoptysis.

I   This is presentation of pulmonary tuberculosis. Treatment is started empirically if acid-fast bacilli (AFBs) are seen on Ziehl–Neelsen staining. Culture results (which take much longer) can be used to modify therapy if any bacterial resistance to medication is detected.

A 45-year-old man rescued from a mountaineering accident presents with an open fracture of the tibia. He is in severe pain and the lower left limb is cold and pulseless. The muscles of the distal limb are brownish-black in colour.

G   This is a presentation of gas gangrene. *Clostridium perfringens*, which thrives in the relative anaerobic conditions of necrotic tissue, is the most common infecting organism. Gas gangrene may be rapidly lethal as a result of the fact that the toxins may have both local and systemic effects, e.g. α toxin has local lytic effects on erythrocytes, inflammatory and muscle cells, but can also contribute to hypotension. Severe pain is always a prominent feature. There are characteristic changes in the colour of the overlying skin to a blue–black colour and the appearance of blebs that discharge watery fluid and later blood. The classically described crepitus of gas gangrene is a late feature and often masked by the coexistent oedema.
Gas gangrene is a medical and surgical emergency requiring surgical débridement (amputation is sometimes indicated) and appropriate antibiotic therapy to cover both aerobic and anaerobic organisms.

A 41-year-old sewer worker presents with fever, jaundice and reddened conjunctivae.

A   This is a presentation of leptospirosis which is a zoonosis caused by infection with the Gram-negative bacterium *Leptospira interrogans*. Although commonly referred to as Weil's disease, the latter term was actually used to describe the clinical presentation of jaundice, renal failure and haemorrhage (pulmonary haemorrhage in the original description). This is a severe presentation carrying a 10 per cent mortality rate. In reality there is a wide variation in severity and many cases are probably not diagnosed.
There are two phases of infection: an initial acute phase and a secondary immune phase.
The first phase of infection is characterized by symptoms associated with proliferation and invasion of the leptospires (e.g. fever, headache, reddened conjunctivae). The second phase is characterized by rising antibody titres, with aseptic meningitis being a common finding. It is during this immune phase that jaundice, hepatomegaly and renal failure may develop, resulting in Weil's disease.
Leptospires are sensitive to penicillin treatment.

A 12-year-old boy presents a few days after a sore throat with a punctate, erythematous generalized rash that spares his face. He has a 'strawberry tongue'.

F   This is presentation of scarlet fever caused by the erythrogenic toxin of group A streptococcal infection. This condition usually occurs in young children because by the age of 12 years most individuals have developed antibody against the exotoxin. The tonsils and pharynx are the usually the primary focus of group A streptococcal infection. Release of erythrogenic toxin causes the development of the generalized erythematous macular rash. The punctate lesions are typically accentuated in the skin folds, e.g. axillae, inguinal regions. Strawberry tongue and circumoral pallor are common features of scarlet fever.

98 Medical emergencies

Answers: M F B H C

A 40 year old rescued from a factory fire presents with stridor and cyanosis. Endotracheal intubation is unsuccessful.

M   Cricothyroidotomy is an emergency airway procedure that should be performed only when other means of establishing an airway, including endotracheal intubation, have failed. In this particular case the upper airway obstruction is probably caused by extensive oropharyngeal oedema from inhalation burns. The cricothyroid membrane can be located by feeling for the thyroid cartilage anteriorly (most prominent cartilage of the neck), and then running the index finger down until you can feel a space between the thyroid (superior) and cricoid (inferior) cartilage.

A 21-year-old man presents with status epilepticus.

F   You must check to make sure that the patient is not hypoglycaemic. The seizure may be stopped with intravenous diazepam, and prophylactic phenytoin may be given to prevent further seizures.
In established status epilepticus, intravenous phenytoin is indicated to prevent further seizures. If the seizures continue, general anaesthetic induction agents, e.g. propofol, may be required.

A 35-year-old builder is brought to A&E after suffering a blow to the side of the head at work. He did not lose consciousness but 4 hours afterwards complained of a severe headache. He became very confused and his conscious level is deteriorating. On examination he has a dilated right pupil. Pulse 50 beats/min, BP 168/100 mmHg.

B   Given the history of head injury and signs of raised intracranial pressure, it is likely that there is an extradural haemorrhage. This is usually caused by a skull fracture tearing the middle meningeal artery. In this particular scenario, the patient is displaying a Cushing response (dropping pulse and rising blood pressure) with a lateralizing sign (dilated right pupil), and there is a high risk of coning. Emergency management involves drilling a Burr hole, evacuating the haematoma and clipping the middle meningeal artery to stem the bleeding.

A 30-year-old woman is rushed to A&E after a stab wound to the chest. On examination her heart sounds are muffled and the JVP rises on inspiration. BP 75/40 mmHg.

H   Hypotension, muffled heart sounds and a JVP that rises on inspiration after chest trauma suggest acute cardiac tamponade.
Emergency pericardiocentesis is indicated to drain the build-up of pericardial fluid, which is preventing the heart from filling.

A 34-year-old woman collapses at the airport arrivals lounge with sudden dyspnoea. BP 90/42 mmHg, Pao_2 6.0 kPa.

C   The low systolic blood pressure and hypoxia suggest significant compromise. Oxygen, intravenous fluids and insulin are indicated as first-line management. There is increasing evidence that thrombolysis improves outcome in large pulmonary emboli. In patients who do not respond to drug therapy, open surgical embolectomy may be indicated as a last resort.

99 The confused patient

Answers: M G J N H

A 53-year-old man presents to A&E confused and unsteady on his feet. On examination he has nystagmus and bilateral lateral rectus palsies. He smells strongly of alcohol.

M   Wernicke's encephalopathy is at the top of the differential diagnosis list and so administering thiamine is a priority to avoid progression to irreversible Korsakoff's syndrome.

A 28-year-old woman presents confused and weak after collapsing in the street. Examination reveals tachycardia, marked hypotension and several depigmented patches over her body. Hb 14 g/dl, BM 3.5 mmol/l, serum Na^+ 128 mmol/l, serum K^+ 5.4 mmol/l, serum Ca^{2+} 2.6 mmol/l.

G   This is a presentation of an addisonian crisis. The patient may have Addison's disease or may have suddenly stopped taking long-term steroid treatment. Intravenous hydrocortisone sodium succinate is the initial treatment of choice. The patient is often hypoglycaemic and so this should also be treated as required. Fludrocortisone may be required long term.

A 15-year-old boy presents acutely confused with hyperventilation, vomiting and abdominal pain. Hb 14 g/dl, white cell count 13.0×10^9/l, BM 19 mmol/l, platelets 160×10^9/l.

J   This is a presentation of diabetic ketoacidosis (a medical emergency) for which fluids are the single most important therapeutic measure.
The dehydration is a more severe complication than the prevailing hyperglycaemia.

A 73-year-old woman with a history of metastatic breast cancer presents with vomiting and abdominal pain. She is found to be acutely confused. On examination positive findings include dry mucous membranes. Hb 10 g/dl, white cell count 7×10^9/l, BM 4.5 mmol/l, platelets 350×10^9/l, corrected calcium 4.2 mmol/l, serum K^+ 3.5 mmol/l.

N   This is an emergency presentation of hypercalcaemia. In a patient of this age and history, the cause is probably malignancy.
Intravenous saline is an important first-line measure to rehydrate the patient and to increase renal loss of calcium. Intravenous bisphosphonates, e.g. pamidronate, are indicated to lower the serum calcium over a few days.

A 26-year-old woman presents with fever, confusion and agitation. Examination reveals an irregular pulse of rate about 240/min and the presence of a goitre.

H   This is a presentation of a thyroid crisis also known as a thyrotoxic storm. The symptoms are that of hyperthyroidism but more severe. Precipitating factors include recent thyroid surgery, radioiodine therapy, infection and stress.
As a result of the extreme hypermetabolic state, the priorities of management are rehydration and cooling with intravenous fluids. The next priority is to block the peripheral action of the hormone and reduce synthesis of hormone using β blockers, e.g. propranolol and antithyroid drugs, e.g. carbimazole, respectively.

100 Drugs and immunity

Answers: I M J D E

A 28-year-old man requires medication to prevent kidney transplant rejection.

I   Ciclosporin and tacrolimus are the mainstay of chronic anti-rejection therapy. Ciclosporin is a toxic drug with a narrow therapeutic index. Nephrotoxicity is the most common serious complication and both therapeutic plasma monitoring and monitoring of renal function is indicated. Use of ciclosporin with cytochrome P450 inhibitors will reduce the hepatic clearance of the drug and lead to increased risk of toxicity. Tacrolimus is more potent but also more neurotoxic and nephrotoxic than ciclosporin.

A 35-year-old man reports being bitten by a bat while on holiday abroad a few weeks ago.

M   In this patient, post-exposure rabies immunization is indicated.
Rabies is a rhabdovirus with a marked affinity for salivary glands (hence transfer through biting) and nervous tissue. The incubation period can be up to 3 months and so it is not uncommon for there to be a long period

of time elapsing between transfer of infection and onset of symptoms. The classic form of rabies is known as 'furious rabies'.

Symptoms in the prodromal period include fever, malaise, headache and itching at the site of the bite. The patient may become agitated, hallucinate and exhibit bizarre behaviour. The patient should be nursed in a quiet, darkened room because the hallmark of furious rabies is hyperexcitability to auditory and visual stimulation. Hydrophobia is present as a result of severe pharyngeal spasm when the patient attempts to eat or drink. Death is inevitable once the classic signs appear.

A 21-year-old man returning from a camping holiday presenting with diplopia and photophobia develops cardiorespiratory failure.

J   This is the presentation of botulism. It should be remembered that the symptoms occur with no gastrointestinal signs. There is marked cholinergic blockade. Respiratory insufficiency can be considerable and therefore there should be no delay in intubating patients if it is deemed necessary.

A 40-year-old woman with multiple sclerosis (MS) is prescribed medication to reduce the number of relapses.

D   Interferon-β has been shown to reduce the number of plaques/lesions seen on magnetic resonance imaging (MRI) over time in patients with MS. Patients should be referred to a neurologist to establish whether treatment is indicated.

Interferon-α is indicated in chronic hepatitis C infection.

A 30-year-old woman presents with a laceration on her hand sustained while gardening. She has not had any injections in the last 15 years.

E   Post-exposure prophylaxis with tetanus immunization is indicated. Tetanus vaccine stimulates the production of protective antitoxin.

The infective agent responsible is *Clostridium tetani*, the spores of which are often found in soil. Pathology results from the release of an exotoxin. The neurotoxin responsible (tetanospasmin) causes disinhibition at motor synapses and promotes neuromuscular blockade, giving rise to the characteristic skeletal muscle spasm. The most obvious sign of generalized tetanus is the appearance of 'lockjaw' (trismus caused by masseter muscle spasm). Facial muscle spasm gives rise to the characteristic risus sardonicus (grinning expression). Progressive muscle spasm causes arching of the neck and back muscles (opisthotonus). Laryngeal spasm impairs ventilation and can be life threatening.

The patient usually presents with non-specific symptoms of fever, headache and general malaise before the onset of the classic pathognomonic signs. Active immunization with tetanus toxoid is given along with pertussis and diphtheria vaccine during the first year of life. Boosters are given before school/nursery school entry and in early adulthood. In this scenario tetanus immunization should be administered because more than 10 years have elapsed since the previous booster.

Index

Note: Numbers refer to Questions not pages. Numbers preceded by 'Box' refer to Revision Boxes, thus 'Box 6.2' is Revision Box 2 in Section 6